Antigenic Determinants and Immune Regulation

Chemical Immunology

(formerly 'Progress in Allergy')

Vol. 46

KARGER

Basel · München · Paris · London · New York · New Delhi · Bangkok · Singapore · Tokyo · Sydney

Antigenic Determinants and Immune Regulation

Volume Editor
Eli Sercarz, Los Angeles, Calif.

23 figures and 23 tables, 1989

KARGER

Basel · München · Paris · London · New York · New Delhi · Bangkok · Singapore · Tokyo · Sydney

Chemical Immunology

Formerly published as 'Progress in Allergy'
Founded 1939 by *Paul Kallós*, Helsingborg

Bibliographic Indices
This publication is listed in bibliographic services, including Current Contents® and Index Medicus.

Drug Dosage
The authors and the publisher have exerted every effort to ensure that drug selection and dosage set forth in this text are in accord with current recommendations and practice at the time of publication. However, in view of ongoing research, changes in government regulations, and the constant flow of information relating to drug therapy and drug reactions, the reader is urged to check the package insert for each drug for any change in indications and dosage and for added warnings and precautions. This is particularly important when the recommended agent is a new and/or infrequently employed drug.

Printed in Switzerland by Thür AG Offsetdruck, Pratteln
ISBN 3-8055-4960-1

Contents

Preface

As this series approaches its 50th anniversary volume, it is instructive to look back half that time to 1963 when it was not known whether separate T-cell subpopulations existed, and when the difference between the specificity of delayed type hypersensitivity and antibodies was first becoming apparent. The thymus had just been shown to be influential in the immune response and the essential feature of T-cell specificity, major histocompatibility complex (MHC) restriction, was not to be learned for another 10 years. The profound effect of the MHC is an overriding influence whose structural basis has only recently been learned from crystallographic studies and whose functional role in binding antigenic peptides has concurrently been revealed.

In this volume, the specificities of T and B lymphocytes are compared with emphasis on the diversity of recognition of MHC molecules and nominal antigens. In this survey we include recognition of hapten, MHC molecules, self-antigens, T-suppressor-, T-helper- and cytotoxic T-cell-inducing determinants, contrasting where possible the variety and distinctions between different cell subpopulations. Furthermore, some general principles of regulation and organization in the immune system are presented in a number of the articles.

The first article by Joel Goodman addresses very generally the structural requirements for antigenicity and immunogenicity at both the T- and B-cell levels. The nature of protein determinants for each subpopulation of lymphocytes is compared, and the author's own extensive studies on the unusual haptenic T-cell determinant, *L*-tyrosine-*p*-azobenzenearsonate are described. The presentation of the material is within the context of the very current paradigms on detailed class-II structure (derived from the studies of class-I MHC crystals). After describing the conceptual basis of determinant structure, relevant examples are provided in vaccine models for the rational application of these principles to actual immunization.

The next two articles provide an up-to-the-minute assessment of MHC class-I and II structures and their influence on immune recognition. Through the use of variant MHC molecules, either by mutation of one or a few amino acids, or through genetic engineering (interchange of exons), effects can then be studied on the conservation of determinants recognized by T cells or by antibodies. Both articles conclude that antigen-specific T cells recognize amino acid residues on the MHC molecule as well as a determinant derived by processing from the nominal antigen. This determinant lies in a cleft, the floor of which consists of β-pleated sheets, flanked by α helices encoded by different domains of the MHC molecules. In the recognition by alloreactive T cells, it may be that processed self or foreign peptides occupy the cleft. These studies depend very directly on the three-dimensional structural framework provided by the crystallographers, which at least in the class-I molecule, directly locate each residue. Those amino acids located on the α_1 and α_2 helices that have side chains directed upwards or into the antigenic cleft profoundly influence T-cell reactivity. Sometimes even a single amino acid change can exert a potent effect. In the case of the recognition by antibodies, which as might have been expected, concerns superficial residues, the majority of serological epitopes are confined to spatially discrete, individual domains. Bluestone and Potter review studies showing that even residues in α_3 can play a critical role in establishing the functional interaction of the T cell and target cell, if they comprise part of the site recognized by the CD8 molecule.

Since the class-II molecule is an α-β chain heterodimer, polymorphic residues can be identified that are responsible for regulating α/β chain allele-specific association, and others that regulate cell surface expression. As McKean points out, although the three-dimensional details of class-II structure are still unknown, cell-surface expression of the molecule clearly depends on interaction of constituent chains in the floor of the antigen-binding site. Studies on antigen binding to class-II molecules and processing of antigen for class-II association have progressed much further than in the case of class I.

The next three papers explore reactivity to determinants on self antigens. Fritz and McFarlin present a broad historical outline of studies on myelin basic protein, from the perspective of the encephalitogenic response to each of the determinants in different strains, and its regulation. The factors considered are the immunodominance of different determinants, the role of suppressor cells directed against certain sites on myelin basic protein and the comparison between the antibody and T-cell responses. The article by Kapp and Whiteley focuses on the existence of immune responses to autologous proteins such as insulin. Whether tolerance to these self molecules is dependent on clonal deletion or suppressor T cells is considered. What is clearly evident is that qualitatively 'ordinary' T-helper cell memory can be induced to autologous insulin, and that these T-helper cells can generally be revealed by removal of T-suppressor cells.

Accordingly, at least some of the T-cell repertoire remains intact to a variety of self antigens. Another important set of self determinants are idiotopes: Mark Greene and his colleagues investigate the fascinating network implications of their studies in the reovirus system, as well as considering determinants of the virus. The intertwining of viral receptor and anti-idiotypic internal image antibodies in this system serve as a prototype for linkage between physiological receptors and the immune system. In these studies, the internal image anti-idiotype (Ab-2) has sequences which are identical to the reovirus hemagglutinin. Furthermore, within a circumscribed region of the Ab-2 molecule are determinants capable of inducing either T cells or antibody formation.

The last two contributions are overviews of suppression and immunodominance, relating to the factors influencing the outcome of response to a multideterminant antigen. Mitchison has made an intriguing synthesis of a vast amount of information on suppressor T cells. He presents some of his new precepts on cell clusters as organizational units of parallel suppressor cell and helper cell induction and interaction, on the nature of Ir/Is genes and MHC restriction, and the possibility that a single restriction element can be used under certain circumstances for activating T cells of opposite function. Sercarz addresses the problem of why certain determinants 'win out' in immunization with multideterminant antigen. Several aspects are considered with emphasis on topological, architectural aspects of each determinant in the structure: how the tertiary, tightly folded molecule is processed to sequentially reveal the set of determinants that have affinity for MHC molecules is considered a major factor. Two features of intramolecular competition are stressed: (a) how the initial binding of one determinant on the unfolding antigenic molecule to the MHC influences the subsequent pattern of processing and determinant usage, and (b) the relationship between T-suppressor-inducing and T-helper cell-inducing determinants. The point is also made that structural relationships for cellular communication as well as the concentration relationships between antigen and MHC molecule in vivo are quite different from the in vitro situation.

It is hoped that this survey of the universe of 'self' and 'foreign' determinants may serve to blur the distinction between these categories. As network adherents have pointed out, the extracorporeal world of determinants merely contains external images of a much broader universe of internal structures. The importance of self-recognition by T cells is undisputed and in this monograph although the emphasis has been on the diversity of immune recognition, it is clear that the symmetries will soon become increasingly evident.

Eli Sercarz, Editor

Sercarz E (ed): Antigenic Determinants and Immune Regulation. Chem Immunol.
Basel, Karger, 1989, vol 46, pp 1–22

Modelling Determinants for Recognition by B Cells and T Cells

Joel W. Goodman[1]

Department of Microbiology and Immunology, University of California,
San Francisco, Calif., USA

Introduction

This article will address our current understanding of the structural features of antigens, principally protein antigens, which are responsible for *antigenicity* (determinants reactive with antibody) on the one hand and *immunogenicity* (determinants that activate T cells) on the other. This subject is of more than academic interest because it promises rational approaches to the fabrication of synthetic vaccines. It is, of course, now generally appreciated that interaction of antigens with antibodies and T cell receptors is fundamentally different. Antibodies bind antigens directly whereas T cells recognize antigen only in the context of proteins encoded by the major histocompatibility complex (MHC) on antigen-presenting cell (APC) surfaces. This requirement for activation and effector function of T cells, known as MHC restriction, ensures that they interact only with other cells and cannot be diverted by soluble antigen. It also furnishes an explanation for seminal observations [1] on specificity differences between antibodies and T cells, which received abundant confirmation [2–4] and ultimately led to the concept that protein antigens are 'processed' (denatured or degraded) prior to recognition by T cells. The essential tenet that antibodies induced by native proteins react weakly, if at all, with denatured or fragmented antigen, whereas T cells are not only undistracted by antigen manipulation but customarily require it, received its most conclusive experimental verification from the demonstration that a T cell hybridoma

[1] Supported by NIH Grant AI-05664.

responded to a peptide digest of ovalbumin, but not to the native protein, presented by purified Ia in planar membranes [5].

Specificity differences between B and T cells have also been discernible at the epitope level. Guinea pig cellular and humoral responses to bovine glucagon, an immunogenic polypeptide of 29 amino acids, were directed at different regions of the antigen [6]. Similar findings were obtained with hen egg lysozyme (HEL) [7] and, in fact, responses to hapten-carrier conjugates exemplify the distinction between humoral and cellular specificity. Today it is widely believed that haptens, regardless of size, are nonimmunogenic principally because they are unable to form functional complexes with MHC molecules (determinant selection), although gaps in the T cell antigen receptor repertoire may also be responsible in some instances. Direct support for determinant selection models of immune responsiveness came from in vitro demonstration of binding of immunogenic peptides to purified class II MHC molecules [8, 9], the most convincing aspect of which was the conformity to predictions based on Ir gene effects. Thus, the peptides in question bound much better to Ia from responder haplotypes than to nonresponder Ia. Furthermore, experiments with a series of peptides from HEL showed a correlation between the ability of nonimmunogenic peptides to competitively inhibit T cell proliferative responses to the immunogenic peptide, which had been demonstrated earlier in several other systems [10–12], and their capacity to block the in vitro binding of the peptide to Ia [13], thereby establishing a connection between peptide-Ia interaction and the cellular response. These findings were extended and broadened by the demonstration that immunogenic peptides from unrelated antigens competed in T cell activation protocols only if they shared a common MHC restriction [14], implying the existence of a unique, specific site on Ia for ligand interaction, consistent with models of MHC molecules based on X-ray diffraction analysis [15, 16]. Interestingly, a peptide from bacteriophage λ cI repressor bound to I-E^d in a specific manner, but did not give I-E^d-restricted responses [14]. This peptide bore homology at several positions to a polymorphic region of I-E^d itself, affording both an intriguing, albeit unproven, explanation for the unresponsive state on the basis of auto-tolerance, and an example of unresponsiveness likely caused by a gap in the repertoire rather than by determinant selection. An alternative possibility is that the peptide-I-E^d combination elicits a suppressor response similar to that seen with hen egg lysozyme in H-2^b mice [17]. However, proponents of this idea would have to explain why the I-A^d-restricted response is not suppressed in H-2^d mice, and there is no evidence to my knowledge that the effector arm of suppression is locus-specific.

The competitive functional and binding studies support bifunctional models of T cell immunogens [17, 18], which hypothesize distinct sites on the determinant for binding to MHC (agretope) and to the antigen receptor (epitope). This terminology was originally coined by Schwartz and his colleagues [18]. Thus, immunogenic determinants, which are capable of activating T cells, are functionally more complex than antigenic determinants, which simply consist of epitopes reactive with antibodies. Peptides from myoglobin, staphylococcal nuclease and λ repressor giving I-E^d-restricted T cell responses manifest significant sequence homology, suggesting implication of the homologous residues in agretope function [14]. Because the peptides do not cross-stimulate T cells, nonhomologous residues are probably responsible for epitope function. Inasmuch as T cell responses to defined determinants are typically heterogeneous [19–21], suggesting an ample T cell specificity repertoire, agretope function is likely to be response limiting in most instances, although the case of λ repressor and I-E^d cited above is a noteworthy exception. Thus, any modelling of T cell determinants must acknowledge the requirement for dual functional sites.

Finally, this article will only address determinants for class-II-restricted T cells, about which more is known at this point. Class-I- and class-II-restricted T cell antigen recognition appear similar in some important respects [16, 22], but significant differences in antigen processing and presentation to the two T cell types have been reported [23]. In any event, too little is known about the detailed structure of class-I-restricted determinants to justify model building.

Antigenic Determinants

The discrete regions of protein or saccharide antigens (determinants or epitopes) that interact with antibody binding sites (paratopes) have been shown by numerous studies, dating back to the classic work of Kabat [24] on dextrans, to span some 4–7 amino acid or sugar residues in the antigen [reviewed in ref. 25]. The epitopes may consist of a linear sequence of residues, in which case they are called continuous, or residues which are not linearly arranged in the sequence but are brought into juxtaposition by conformational folding, in which case they are called discontinuous, or assembled topographic, epitopes [26].

The number and location of antigenic determinants in proteins has been a subject of substantial controversy, fueled by the limitations of the methods used for epitope mapping. A popular and simple approach has been to test antibodies raised to the native protein for binding to fragments of the protein. The major difficulty here is that most antibodies recognize conformational features of the antigen and react poorly, if at all, with peptide fragments. Differences in binding affinity of antibodies with intact and fragmented antigens vividly underscore this point. Thus, this approach minimizes epitope numbers and probably favors identification of sites with a high degree of mobility, permitting the peptide to bind to at least some of the antibody produced to a flexible segment of the protein.

The converse approach, reacting anti-peptide antibodies with the native protein to draw conclusions about epitope location, poses much the same risk. Again, since the conformation of the peptide coupled to a carrier is likely to differ from that of the homologous sequence in the native protein, antibodies to peptides representing regions of high flexibility in the protein are likely to cross-react best. It should be appreciated that this method does not map the native epitopes of the protein, but simply discloses whether particular anti-peptide antibodies discernibly react with the protein. However, a body of data obtained with monoclonal anti-protein antibodies argues that most, if not all, of the surface of proteins consists of a series of overlapping epitopes [26]. A persuasive case in point is insulin, a small protein which has induced more than 100 monoclonal antibodies of different specificity [27]. Returning to the reactivity of anti-peptide antibodies with native proteins, a surprisingly large fraction cross-reacted in a study using a series of 20 synthetic peptides representing about 75% of the surface of the influenza hemagglutinin protein [28]. However, binding affinities of the anti-peptide antibodies with protein were not determined and binding was assayed with hemagglutinin adsorbed to a solid surface, which may have caused denaturation [29]. Therefore, issues concerning binding, and relative strength of binding, to truly native protein were not resolved. However, in another study with myohemerythrin, one monoclonal antibody was obtained to a synthetic peptide that apparently reacted better with soluble protein than with the peptide itself, although reactivity with the apoprotein was better still [30], indicating that relaxation of the native conformation improved binding. In any case, reports of such heteroclitic activity are relatively rare, which bears on the subject of synthetic vaccines to be considered later.

Peptide reactivity with anti-protein antibodies has been used to map a limited number of immunodominant regions on about a dozen structurally defined proteins. Bearing in mind the limitations of the approach, these regions represent continuous epitopes which have been used in attempts to decipher the relationship between protein structure and antigenicity. This subject has been reviewed elsewhere [26, 31] and only a few relevant points will be made here. The data have been analyzed for correlations between epitope location and such parameters as hydrophilicity, surface accessibility (which should correlate closely with hydrophilicity), segmental flexibility or mobility, amphipathicity, protrusion and chain termination. Unsurprisingly, the best correlation has been with mobility, but the method, based on reactivity of anti-protein antibodies with small peptides, is biased in its favor. Indeed, there is no prima facie evidence that mobile regions of proteins are preferentially immunodominant and, in fact, the use of longer peptides can reveal epitopes in regions of low mobility [31], presumably because longer peptides can better mimic local conformation in the protein. Throw in the considerations that space-filling models of proteins show that most of the surface is dictated by polypeptide chain folding and that most monoclonal anti-protein antibodies are directed against discontinuous determinants [26], and it becomes apparent that epitope mapping by peptide reactivity reveals only a fraction of the whole.

Thus, the tenets of antigenicity remain elusive, but at least one principle should be clear. If a peptide is employed to generate anti-protein antibodies, the best bet would be a sequence from a surface region with a high degree of mobility in the protein. This should maximize prospects for cross-reactivity of the anti-peptide antibody.

Immunogenic Determinants

In contrast to B cell epitopes, which are largely discontinuous and may blanket the entire surface of a protein antigen, determinants recognized by T cells are more restricted in location and are usually defined by a linear array of amino acids in the protein sequence. As alluded to above, the constraints on T cell determinants are largely dictated by the requirement for functionally relevant association with MHC molecules rather than by gaps in the T cell specificity repertoire. Thus, there has been substantial interest in defining the properties of T cell determinants, with the goal of understanding the common structural denominator, if such exists, responsible for conferring the recondite quality we call 'immunogenicity'.

The principal strategy for identifying T cell determinants of proteins is much like that used to map antigenic determinants, utilizing fragments of the proteins to assess T cell responses. Sets of synthetic peptide analogs of an active fragment are then used to more precisely map the immunogenic determinant. Stimulatory peptides are seldom shorter than a decamer, although some noteworthy exceptions will be discussed further. In an evaluation of the effect of peptide length on stimulatory activity, T cell lines specific for a determinant of cytochrome *c* could respond to a decapeptide, but maximal stimulation required a 16mer [32, 33], suggesting the possibility that the additional residues stabilized a particular secondary structure [34]. The question of conformational requirements for immunogenicity will be considered in more detail later. A priori, it seems logical that immunogenic determinants might exceed antigenic determinants in size. First, the immunogenic determinant must include both agretope and epitope. Second, the antigen-binding sites of T cell receptors and antibodies are similar in organization and may accommodate epitopes of comparable dimension. However, an unknown here is how much of the binding site is devoted to MHC restriction, so the jury is still out on this one.

The exceptional immunogenic determinants referred to above are *L*-tyrosine-*p*-azobenzenearsonate (ABA-Tyr) [35], hepta-*L*-lysine [36], which is immunogenic in strain 2 guinea pigs, and angiotensin II octapeptides [37], also stimulatory in guinea pigs. Whether these, and particularly ABA-Tyr (only 409 daltons), induce T cell responses by the same mechanism as larger peptides is still open to question. However, it has been shown that ABA-D-Tyr is nonimmunogenic, as is a sequence of fewer than seven residues of the *L* isomer of lysine. Therefore, it seems unlikely, but not impossible, that they act indirectly by associating with endogenous peptides which, in turn, associate with Ia. It may also be significant that these smaller determinants seem to be more active in guinea pigs than mice, although even ABA-Tyr is weakly immunogenic in mice. The angiotensin octapeptides do not evoke a detectable response in mice [Thomas, personal communication]. Perhaps the likeliest explanation for the apparent differences relates to sensitivity of the two species to the assays used for detecting responses, but subtle differences in antigen processing could also be responsible.

About 50 peptides housing class-II-restricted immunogenic determinants have been described as of this writing, and the list steadily grows. A compendium of class-I-restricted and class-II-restricted T cell peptide determinants has been published recently [38] and is nearly up to date. Detailed studies of the responses to these determinants have revealed a number of telling facets of T cell antigen recognition.

(1) T cell responses to individual determinants are generally heterogeneous, reflecting the recruitment of multiple T cell differing in fine specificity for the nominal antigen. This is true even for a determinant as small as ABA-Tyr [19] and has been repeatedly demonstrated for larger peptide determinants [39, 40]. The diversity of responses to limited epitopes argues strongly for an abundant T cell specificity repertoire and for limitations imposed on T cell antigen recognition by other parameters, such as the disposition of functional agretopes. A large specificity repertoire is consistent with analyses of the numbers and rearrangement patterns of T cell receptor genes, despite the apparent absence of somatic mutation as a deversification mechanism [41].

(2) Determinant selection shows a striking class II locus and allele preference in mice. Data for other species is insufficient to permit conclu-

sions. Particular determinants from the same protein may preferentially associate with either I-A or I-E for antigen presentation. Thus, a determinant in a peptide spanning residues 106–118 of sperm whale myoglobin is I-A^d-restricted, whereas a second determinant from residues 132–146 is E^d-restricted [42]. Analogous situations have been demonstrated for responses to HEL [43] and the cytochromes [44]. There are numerous examples of allele preference at a given locus [see ref. 38 for a compilation] and this propensity is clearly germane to Ir gene defects. In the response to ABA-Tyr, only I-A-restricted clones were obtained from mice which were non-b (the only low responder phenotype to this immunogen) at the A locus [45–47]. However, B10.A(5R) mice, which are I-A^b but E^k_α, yielded E-restricted clones [45], demonstrating that this determinant could be presented by I-E as well as I-A, although a strong preference for the latter was apparent.

(3) Although most clonal T cell responses are rigidly MHC-restricted, that is, the antigen is recognized only in context of syngeneic Ia, MHC degeneracy has been observed in some responses [40, 44, 45, 48]. In the majority of instances where antigen can be presented by allo-MHC, the responses have been I-E-restricted [40, 44, 45]. However, degeneracy in the I-A-restricted response to a determinant from pigeon cytochrome *c* has been reported [48]. Nevertheless, the association of degeneracy with I-E restriction seems unlikely to be random or trivial. In the response to ABA-Tyr, none of more than 20 I-A^k-restricted clones from A/J and B10.A(2R) mice were found to be degenerate, whereas 4 of 10 I-E-restricted clones from B10.A(5R) mice were [45]. The degenerate clones responded to APC from k or d haplotype mice as well as to syngeneic feeders. E_α k and d alleles differ by only 3 amino acids and none of the differences are in the first domain [49]. The E_β locus is much more polymorphic [50], with differences between the b, k and d alleles ranging from 7 to 21. The findings suggest, but do not prove, a strong functional role for E_α in antigen recognition by the degenerate clones. In another study, T cells from B10.A(5R) mice responded to either of two determinants from the herpes simplex virus glycoprotein D, one in the context of I-A and the other with I-E [40]. Only the I-E-restricted response was degenerate, and all the clones of this type proved to be so. If the correlation of MHC degeneracy with I-E is real, it may be related to the limited polymorphism of E_α. An intriguing facet of degeneracy is the influence of the Ia molecule on the fine specificity of the T cell response [40, 44]. This effect can be interpreted as due to differences in the way the nominal determinant sits in the binding site of different Ia molecules, or to variations of a complex determinant comprised of contributions from the nominal epitope and from Ia. In any event, it is clear that Ia structure profoundly affects T cell specificity.

Functional Substructure and Structural Motifs of Immunogenic Determinants

Components of T cell determinants that contribute to class II binding and to epitope configuration have been tentatively identified using analogs of the determinant in question. Nonstimulatory compounds that retain binding with class II protein, assessed either by direct binding to purified protein or indirectly by their capacity to block presentation of the parent determinant to T cells, are assumed to possess intact agretopes but deficient epitopes. Conversely, substitutions or deletions causing loss of binding or blocking activity are interpreted as agretopic sites. The first immunogenic determinant to be scrutinized by this type of analysis was the nonpeptide compound ABA-Tyr. It was found early on that substituents at the arsonate position dictated T cell specificity without necessarily affecting immunogenicity [35], implicating the arsonate moiety in the epitope. A series of nonstimulatory analogs of ABA-Tyr were later used to block presentation of the immunogenic compound in an effort to define the agretope [10]. Compounds bearing the azo-linked aromatic ring structure blocked presentation of ABA-Tyr in a dose-dependent way, whereas a mixture of *p*-arsanilic acid and *L*-tyrosine was ineffective. The blocking pattern given by the family of analogs indicated that agretope function centered on the azo-linked aromatic rings, with little or no contribution from either the arsonate group or the tyrosyl side chain. On the other hand, T cell clones segregated in their capacity to recognize analogs with modified tyrosyl side chains, suggesting that the side chain contributed to the epitope of ABA-Tyr and that different clones manifested different fine specificities for the nominal determinant, a common feature of T cell responses noted above. Some clones also responded to one of the two isomers of ABA-histidine (4-ABA-His), but not to the other (2-ABA-His). 4-ABA-His blocked the presentation of ABA-Tyr to clones unresponsive to the His compound, further supporting the presence of an agretope in this molecule. Computer modelling of ABA-Tyr and the two isomers of ABA-His revealed that the alpha carbon backbones of ABA-Tyr and 4-ABA-His lie in the same plane relative to the azo linkage, whereas the backbone of nonstimulatory 2-ABA-His is in the opposite orientation. All these findings are compatible with the hypothesis that this class of compounds binds to class II proteins through its azo-linked ring structure, which orients the arsonate and amino acid side chain moieties to form the epitope recognized by the T cell. A conspicuous property of the putative agretope is its hydrophobicity, whereas the subregions comprising the putative epitope are strongly hydrophilic. As we shall see, there is substantial evidence that this comprises a favored motif for T cell determinants.

Berzofsky has championed the hydrophobic agretope-hydrophilic epitope concept by calling attention to the amphipathic character of a major proportion of immunogenic peptide determinants from protein antigens [42]. This story began with a detailed analysis of a determinant spanning residues 132–146 of sperm whale myoglobin, which is in an α-helical configuration in the native protein [reviewed in ref. 42]. The possible significance of helices for immunogenicity was originally noted by Pincus et al. [34] in the pigeon cytochrome system referred to earlier. Using a series of truncated and substituted myoglobin peptides, four residues critical for T cell activation were identified. All four were charged and positioned on the solvent-exposed face of the helix. The other side of the helix, composed of hydrophobic residues, is buried in the protein, which Berzofsky and colleagues reasoned could explain the requirement for processing of the protein, but not of the peptide, on the basis that the hydrophobic face was also essential for T cell activation. They concluded that one face might interact with the T cell receptor and the other with the class II MHC molecule. Noting that another myoglobin determinant exhibited the same properties, they reasoned that amphipathic helices may have an advantage in determinant selection, aided, perhaps, by their facility for intercalating into cell membranes, thereby attaining high local concentrations which should favor MHC association [42]. Accordingly, they developed a computer program to identify amphipathic segments on the basis of primary structure and proceeded to analyze known immunogenic peptides. Of 44 known class-II-restricted immunogenic peptides, about 70% can be folded as amphipathic α helices; the corresponding p value is 0.003 [Berzofsky, personal communication]. Furthermore, the algorithm has had predictive value for identifying potential immunogenic sites in proteins. For example, a potential determinant was identified in sperm whale myoglobin and later verified experimentally [39, 42].

Another motif, based strictly on recurring similarities in the primary sequences of immunogenic peptides, has been reported by Rothbard and Taylor [38]. They noted that 46 of 57 class-I- and class-II-restricted peptides contain a sequence of four residues composed of a charged amino acid or a glycine followed by two hydrophobic residues and ending with a polar residue or glycine. Their analysis showed that the probability of this motif occuring in a random 15-residue peptide was 33% as compared to the actual occurrence of 81% in the immunogenic peptides, yielding a p value of less than 0.001. The four-residue pattern has been identified in helical segments and in β strands of proteins with known three-dimensional structure. However, the conformation of the segment in the native protein may be immaterial inasmuch as the T cell sees a processed peptide. Therefore, the conformation of the peptide itself should dictate association with MHC to form an immunogenic determinant. In this context, it may be of interest that the four-residue sequences can be modelled as one turn of an amphiphatic α helix [42].

It should be noted that there are bonafide immunogenic peptides that are not predicted by either the amphipathic or the four-residue cassette algorithms, as reflected by their 70–80% success rates. Indeed, the two-peptide determinants that have been extensively mapped for agretope and epitope subregions, HEL 52–61 [51] and ovalbumin 325–335 [52], though each contains a cassette, are dubious candidates for amphipathic α helices. The HEL peptide is simply not amphipathic, though it can be modelled as an α helix [51]. The ovalbumin peptide has predictive amphipathic structure, but based on mapping putative contact sites for Ia and the T cell receptor, it was concluded that the peptide assumes an extended conformation to permit shared recognition of some residues [52]. The validity of this conclusion, based on the effect of amino acid substitutions on Ia binding and on T cell activation, is obviously open to some question. Regardless of the discrepant examples, it is difficult to argue with the general observation that immunogenic determinants tend to share identifiable structural features related to a segregation of hydrophobic and hydrophilic sites, with the potential to form amphipathic secondary structures conferring a selective advantage. This would seemingly relate to the structures of the peptide binding sites on class I [15] and class II [16] molecules, which have β-pleated floors and helical walls, but precisely how it relates is still obscure. The proposed similarity of the two binding sites is also consistent with the parallel properties noted thus far for class-I- and class-II-restricted immunogenic determinants [38, 42].

Where do the azo-linked aromatic compounds fit into this overall scheme? ABA-Tyr clearly has segregated hydrophobic and hydrophilic subregions, as discussed above. If the arsonate moiety and tyrosyl side chain project in the same direction from the plane of the aromatic core, it can readily be visualized that they form an epitope, or part of a complex epitope that includes residues from the helical walls of the class II binding site, which is perceived differently by different T cell receptors, accounting for the observed spectrum of fine specificities. It might be expected that the azo-linked rings would have relatively few contact points with the class II binding site (desetope) compared to the much larger peptide determinants that have been studied, resulting in relatively weak agretope-desetope interaction. This, indeed, is consistent with the relatively weak immunogenicity of ABA-Tyr and with the high concentrations of the compound required for T cell activation (0.1–0.5 mM). In preliminary studies of competitive blocking of the presentation of ABA-Tyr by I-A^k-restricted peptides, an undecapeptide determinant from rat myelin basic protein proved to be 2–3 orders of magnitude more efficient that phenyl-azo-tyrosine on a molar basis [unpublished observations], supporting the weak agretope hypothesis. Additional support derives from the inability of phenyl-azo-tyrosine to block presentation of HEL to an HEL-specific T cell clone [10], which at the time was interpreted as suggesting the existence of multiple desetopes on class II molecules.

Several other observations which initially seemed anomalous are also consonant with weak agretopic function of ABA-Tyr. One was a study of the binding of fluorescein derivatized ABA-Tyr, which can block the presentation of the parent compound and thus retains agretope activity, to I-A protein in artificial planar membranes, a technique which has detected binding of immunogenic peptides [5]. Binding of Flu-ABA-Tyr was undetectible at either pH 7 or pH 5 [McConnell, personal communication], the latter being used to mimic an endosomal environment. Inasmuch as both the crystallographic data for class I molecules [15] and kinetic studies of the association and dissociation of peptide ligands with class II molecules [14] indicate that the binding sites of MHC molecules are normally occupied, a weak agretope should be relatively inefficient at displacing a stronger one. According to this scenario, ABA-Tyr at usable concentrations (up to 0.5 m*M*) might not successfully compete for occupied sites. Furthermore, we have unexpectedly found that chloroquine blocks the presentation of ABA-Tyr, a finding confirmed by Leskowitz [personal communication] who obtained similar results with ammonium chloride and monensin, a carboxylic ionophore that inhibits intracellular trafficking. These agents usually block the presentation of native proteins but not peptide determinants; chloroquine and NH_4Cl are thought to act by inhibiting antigen processing through raising the pH of endosomal and lysosomal compartments in the presenting cell [53]. Small peptides do not usually require processing and hence are unaffected by the agents. On the basis of size alone, ABA-Tyr should segregate with the peptides. However, 'processing' of ABA-Tyr may be needed for presentation because it may be able to complex with class II molecules only in acidic intracellular compartments under conditions where the class II binding site is unoccupied. While the experimental results in the ABA-Tyr system are explicable in terms of weak agretope activity, this remains to be firmly established. What they do suggest is that ABA-Tyr behaves like a conventional immunogenic determinant in the sense that it is presented to T cells by the same class II site that presents peptides such as the myelin basic protein undecamer.

A recently published hypothetical model of the class II antigen-binding site [16] suggests possible contact points for ABA-Tyr. The model predicts that 5 residues from the B_1 domain (Tyr_{30}, Ile_{31}, Tyr_{32}, Tyr_{37} and Val_{38}) lie in close proximity on the β-pleated floor of the binding site (fig. 1), forming

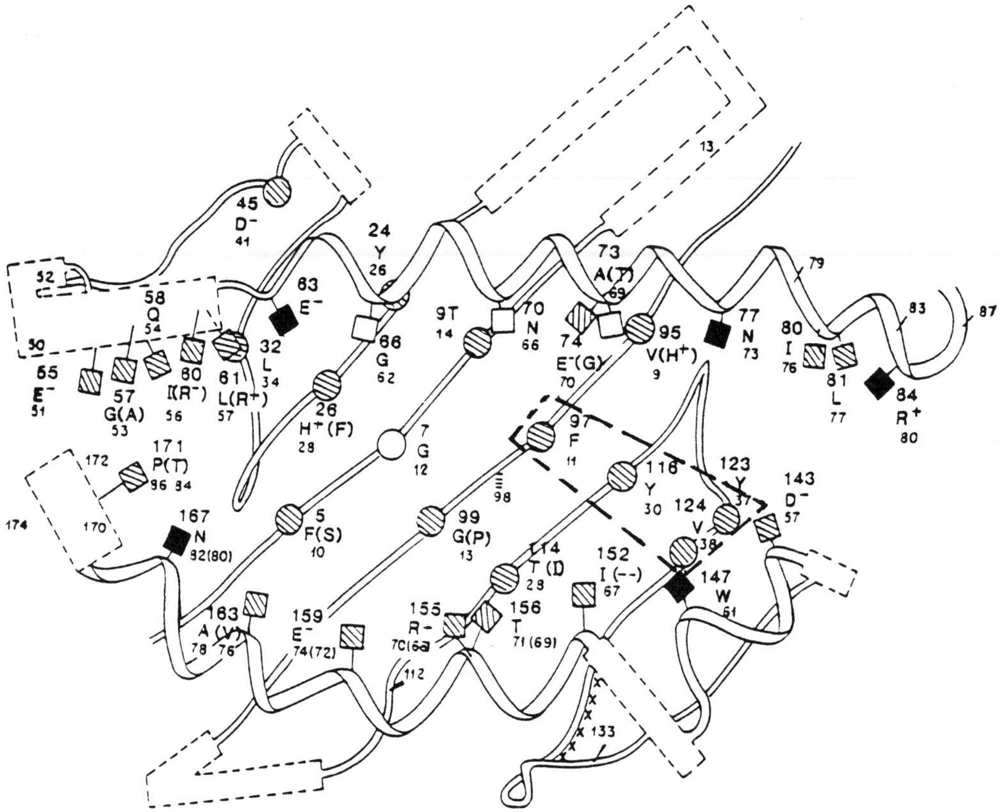

Fig. 1. Hypothetical model of the I-A antigen-binding site as depicted in ref. [16]. The β-pleated floor of the site is flanked by the α (above) and β (below) chain helical segments. Only amino acid residues with side chains projecting into the binding site are shown: squares for residues in helices and circles for those in β-pleated strands. Numbering: bold, HLA-A2; regular, I-A^d; parentheses, I-A^k. For a more complete explanation, see ref. [16]. Reprinted by permission from Nature, vol. 332, No. 6167, p. 849, 1988 ©, MacMillan Journals Limited.

a hydrophobic patch which could anchor ABA-Tyr (or hydrophobic agretopes in general) in the site. Phe_{11}, on the adjacent β strand, is another possible hydrophobic contact point in this extended region. The side chains of the residues at positions 11, 30, 37 and 38 extend into the binding site cavity and thus are depicted within the dashed box in figure 1; amino acids which point in other directions, such as Ile_{31} and Tyr_{32}, are not shown. If the model is substantially correct, only the residues shown project into the binding site and furnish contact points for determinants. Furthermore, Tyr_{30} Tyr_{37} and Val_{38} are positioned relatively near the helical wall of the site contributed by the β chain, suggesting that, if this scenario is correct, polymorphic residues in the β chain helix might contribute to the complex epitope recognized by the T cell. The significance of the β chain in A^k-restricted T cell recognition of ABA-Tyr is discussed below. Conversely, Ile_{31} and Tyr_{32} reside close to the α chain helical segment and do not face into the binding site. Earlier studies with bifunctional antigens composed of two ABA-Tyr units separated by flexible or rigid spacers signified the occurrence of intramolecular ring stacking in the flexibly spaced molecules [35], which essentially reflects hydrophobic interaction between the aromatic rings in the subunits. The evidence from those studies also indicated that interactions between electropositive and electronegative groups in the subunits strongly infuenced stacking. Nonetheless, analogous intermolecular interactions between the aromatic rings of ABA-Tyr and one or more of the aromatic residues on the floor of the binding site could conceivably account for the immunogenicity of this class of compounds. In any case, several other considerations indirectly support the relevance of hydrophobicity in this region to desetope function.

(1) Hydrophobicity at the six positions in question is conserved in all A_β haplotypes that have been sequenced, although conservative substitutions are found in some alleles [54]. In A^q, Tyr_{37} is replaced by Trp, an aromatic hydrophobic substitution, and Phe_{11} is replaced by Leu, an aliphatic, hydrophobic amino acid. Some alleles have Leu instead of Val at position 38, which mildly enhances the hydrophobic character of the region. Thus, hydrophobicity is a general feature of this region in all known I-A molecules, and ABA-Tyr is immunogenic in all mouse strains we have tested [17]. The hydrophobic patch does not explain the weaker responsiveness of $H\text{-}2^b$ mice to ABA-Tyr, since A^b_β has the same hydrophobic alignment in that region as the high responder haplotypes. The only position in A_β which is uniquely b (different from all other haplotypes) is residue 47, where b has His and all other haplotypes have Tyr. His is less hydrophobic than Tyr and position 47 should lie in the β-pleated sheet close to the helical wall of the β_1 domain, according to the model of the class II binding site (fig. 1). If and how this substitution relates to lower responsiveness of $H\text{-}2^b$ is unknown.

(2) An investigation of the presentation of ABA-Tyr to $I\text{-}A^k$-restricted cloned T cells by L cells transfected with class II genes of the k or u haplotype [55] showed that $A^k_\alpha A^k_\beta$(kk) and $A^u_\alpha A^k_\beta$(uk) transfectants were equally effective, whereas the ku and uu transfectants were completely ineffective. The findings indicated that the α chains are interchangeable for activation of ABA-Tyr specific T cells, whereas the β chains are not, a conclusion further supported by subsequent experiments with $A^d_\alpha A^k_\beta$ hybrid transfectants and with hemi-exon shuffled and site-directed mutants of the

β chain gene [56]. Although the configuration of the hydrophobic residues is present in all sequenced β chains, the complex epitope recognized by T cells is likely to vary, depending on particular polymorphic residues in the helical walls of the binding site, accounting for MHC restriction. While detailed conclusions concerning the relative roles of particular Ia sites in T cell recognition is not possible with this approach, the results do suggest that the β chain plays a more critical role than the α chain in the presentation of ABA-Tyr, which is clearly consistent with the above scenario for the class II desetope involved in presentation of ABA-Tyr, particularly with respect to the possible involvement of positions 30, 37 and 38, which sit close to the β chain helix. Site-directed mutagenesis at the putative desetope sites could throw more light on this issue. It is noteworthy that polymorphic residues in the α-chain may be more critical for T cell recognition of other I-A^k-restricted determinants [57].

One can also speculate about the structural basis for the preference of I-A to I-E in the presentation of ABA-Tyr. Assuming homology in the configurations of the I-A and I-E binding sites, position 11 in E_β is Tyr in all sequenced haplotypes, but positions 30 and 37 are Arg or Glu and Glu, respectively [54], drastically reducing the hydrophobicity of the homologous region in E_β. However, positions 31, 32 and 33 in E_β are Tyr or Phe, Phe or Ile and Tyr, respectively, yielding a hydrophobic patch with a different orientation relative to the helical walls of the binding site. The corresponding positions in A_β are Ile, Tyr and Asn, respectively, thus providing two hydrophobic residues and one mildly hydrophilic residue in the analogous region of the binding site floor. However, none of these residues project into the binding site [16], so the net result is reduced hydrophobicity of the region within the I-E binding site, furnishing a plausible explanation for I-A preference in the presentation of ABA-Tyr. It, of course, remains to be seen if these differences between the two β chains do, indeed, directly bear on presentation of ABA-Tyr.

Synthetic Antigens Based on the Principles of Determinant Structure

The practical payoff from understanding the structure-function correlates of antigens would be the rational design of synthetic vaccines. Of course, hapten-carrier conjugates, which have a long history of use, can be considered the 'Model As' of synthetic antigens. This simple principle was applied to the induction of protective humoral immunity against a malaria parasite. *P. falciparum*, by coupling a peptide containing a repetitive sequence from the major sporozoite surface antigen (CS protein), serving as a B cell epitope, to nonmalarial proteins which furnished T cell epitopes [reviewed in ref. 42]. Although protective antibodies were generated by these vaccines, they generate neither memory T help specific for the parasite itself, nor effector T cell immunity which may contribute to defense against injection. In order to correct these deficiencies and develop a vaccine that could induce both B and T cell anti-malarial immunity, the CS protein was screened for amphipathic sequences as candidate immunogenic determinants. The best such site, an octadecapeptide (Th2R), was synthesized, coupled to the repetitive B cell epitope, and the conjugate induced humoral and cellular immunity in responder mice [58]. This second generation synthetic vaccine thus represented a vastly streamlined version that possessed the added virtues of eliciting strictly parasite-specific T and B cell responses, a quantum leap in rational vaccine design. The Th2R region of CS proteins embodies two overlapping T cell determinates which unfortunately map to polymorphic regions of the protein, suggesting an immune evasion mechanism used by the parasite [59]. Analogous antigenic variation affecting reactivity with antibody has been reported for malaria [60] and is well known for influenza, trypanasomiasis and, more recently, human immunodeficiency virus (HIV). Such propensity by infectious agents obviously handicaps the development of broadly efficacious vaccines. Parenthetically, it is of interest in the context of the earlier discussion of minimal size for immunogenic determinants that a heptapeptide from Th2R was sufficient to stimulate T cells, thus comprising the smallest natural determinant described to date [59].

Another successful marriage of synthetic T cell and B cell determinants has been reported for the hepatitis B virus [61]. A synthetic 21-residue peptide common to the capsid and envelope proteins served as a T cell activator in H-2^b and H-2^s mice, albeit the two haplotypes recognized distinct regions within the peptide. That peptide was coupled to an octapeptide hapten from the pre-S(2) region of the envelope, and the composite structure elicited T and B cell responses which cross-reacted with the native proteins. Furthermore, the bifunctional immunogen primed helper cells for subsequent antibody responses to the capsid. Representation of the T cell determinant in the envelope as well as in the capsid suggest the possibility of helper memory for anti-envelope antibody responses as well, but this was not assessed experimentally.

In principle, synthetic vaccines composed of a helper T cell determinant and a B cell epitope seem an ideal solution to the safety and economic problems posed by attenuated, inactivated or subunit vaccines [62, 63]. An approach to an AIDS vaccine by the Berzofsky group [64] employed the same strategy they applied to malaria: identification of sequences in the gp120 envelope protein of HIV with a propensity to form amphipathic helices, and synthesis of the corresponding peptides for use as immunogens in mice. A 16-residue peptide raised T cell immunity to gp120 in three of four different MHC haplotypes, further documenting the utility of this approach for identifying potential T cell determinants. However, distinct limitations to the general approach do exist and warrant consideration. One has to do with determinant selection by different MHC haplotypes, a subject discussed earlier and observed again in the murine responses to the CS and HIV peptides. The Th2R octadecapeptide from the malaria CS protein served as a T helper determinant only in I-A^k mice [58]. This is admittedly an extreme case of Ir gene control in that only H-2^b and H-2^k mice strongly respond to the protein [58], but it does underscore the probability that only a fraction of an outbred population will respond to a given determinant. This was clearly the case in a study of cellular responses by humans living in a malaria-endemic region to a series of overlapping peptides spanning the entire CS protein [65]. The most immunodominant peptide scored with cells from only 14 of the 35 individuals tested.

The limitations imposed by Ir gene control may be at least partially overcome by polyvalent vaccines incorporating most or all of the candidate immunogenic determinants as separate peptides or, more problematically, as tandem sequences in a single peptide. The tandem arrangement is more problematical because antigen processing, the second serious limitation to synthetic vaccines, might destroy one or more of the determinants. This limitation also applies, albeit in a less obvious way, to cross-recognition by T cells of any synthetic peptide determinant and determinants generated by the APC. The point here is that antigen processing is unlikely to yield peptides identical to synthetic homologs. Consequently, even though a peptide is demonstrably immunogenic, it is vital to know if the anti-peptide response cross-recognizes the parent protein, or better still, protects against infection, if the peptide is to serve usefully as a vaccine. A case in point was the observation that a number of individuals in the human malaria study [65] showed no lymphocyte reactivity to any of the peptides in the overlapping set of 11-mers, although they had significant antibody titers against a peptide sequence from the CS protein. Lymphocyte reactivity against the whole protein was not assessed, leaving viable a number of alternative explanations which were considered by the authors. The one that is relevant to this discussion is the possibility that the real determinant in the unresponsive subjects was a peptide of a different size, which called forth a set of T cells that failed to recognize any of the test peptides. This can be visualized as modification of the orientation of similar, but unidentical, peptides in the class II binding site, changing the complex epitope recognized by the T cell antigen receptor and consequently recruiting distinct T cell populations. Experimental evidence supporting this view derives from the failure of T cell clones raised against ABA-Tyr to respond to larger compounds containing the homologous structure, such as fluorescein-Tyr-ABA, which are themselves immunogenic [unpublished observations], and from a recent study of the influence of antigen processing on the expression of the T cell repertoire [66]. In that investigation, it was found that a 17-residue peptide contained the major immunodominant determinant for H-2^s mice immunized with equine myoglobin, whereas H-2^k mice made little, if any, response to that region. However, the peptide itself was immunogenic in both haplotypes. Of particular interest, cells from peptide-immune s mice responded to native myoglobin whereas cells from k mice did not. The absence of cross-recognition by k cells was obviously not due to an inability of the peptide to serve as a determinant in that haplotype, but may have resulted from *in vivo* generation of a processed fragment of myoglobin which could bind to A^s, but not to A^k. Indeed, antigen processing could account for many of the putative gaps in the T cell repertoire.

Agretope Engineering

A third generation form of synthetic vaccines is suggested by the plausibility that agretopes and epitopes of immunogenic determinants are separate structural entities and that agretopes play no direct role in T cell specificity, serving only for MHC binding. There are obvious limitations to this simplistic model, but for the moment let us assume that it is valid in a broad sense. This leads to the prospect of separately designing an optimal agretope which would universally bind with high affinity to a conserved desetope in the class II binding site, minimizing Ir gene effects in outbred populations. Since I have postulated that narrowly focused T cell responses are dictated by agretope function of processed antigens rather than by the T cell antigen receptor repertoire, the major constraint on choice of epitopes would be cross-recognition of the natural antigen by cells primed with the engineered vaccine, which poses a serious obstacle to which we will return later.

What are the candidate desetopes in the class II binding site? Assuming the validity of the hypothetical model of the binding site [16], the conserved hydrophobic patch on the floor, outlined in figure 1, springs readily to mind. The patch consists of four hydrophobic residues in the murine A_β chain which face into the site. These positions are less conserved in human class II genes, although most alleles of DQ have hydrophobic residues there. The only hydrophilic substitutions in 15 sequenced DQ_β alleles [54] are Ser at position 30 in two and Asp at position 37 in one. Ser and Asp do not appear together, so all DQ alleles retain a net hydrophobic character in the zone.

As already mentioned, ABA-Tyr is immunogenic in all mouse haplotypes, suggesting interaction with a relatively conserved region of the class II binding site and strenthening the admittedly speculative argument for desetope functional activity of the hydrophobic patch. A complementary ligand based on the topography of the hydrophobic patch could be designed with hydrophobic amino acids separated by spacers which would permit interaction of a given residue in the synthetic agretope with a like residue in the class II hydrophobic patch. For example, positions 11, 30 and 37 are hydrophobic in the seven sequenced A_{β} chains and lie in a linear array on the binding site floor (fig. 1). It would be relatively simple to design an appropriately spaced hydrophobic tripeptide for theoretically optimal hydrophobic interaction with the class II residues. Epitopes for T and B cells, selected from sequences in the natural antigen, could be added, again using spacers as needed. The use and selection of spacers would be dictated by biological tests to determine cross-reactivity of engineered vaccines with the natural antigen.

The major limitation to using a 'shelf reagent universal agretope' for synthetic vaccines is the problem of cross-reactivity with the natural antigen. Even if the designed agretope works in the sense that it confers immunogenicity on synthetic peptides, there are already indications, as discussed above, that orientation of a given epitope may be critical for T cell recognition. It does seem unlikely, at least at this point in time, that a natural agretope-epitope duo could be adequately mimicked by the unnatural agretope-natural epitope combination, particularly if mimicry of an amphipathic α helix is required. The class II binding site is large relative to immunogenic peptides, as indicated by modelling the HEL 46–61 peptide as a helix and placing it in the site [16]. Thus, many orientations of different peptides are theoretically possible, which perhaps contributes to the specificity of T cells since they would see different nominal epitopes in combination with different residues from the class II site. An additional complication is the evidence that, at least for some determinants, individual amino acids may participate in class II binding *and* T cell binding [52].

Thus, the prospects for third generation synthetic vaccines with engineered agretopes seem discouraging at this time. However, the surface of this new science has barely been scratched. Some of the current truisms may turn out to be blatantly wrong and it is difficult to know what the future holds in store.

References

1 Gell, P.G.H.; Benacerraf, B.: Studies of hypersensitivity. II. Delayed hypersensitivity to denatured proteins in guinea pigs. Immunology *2:* 64–70 (1959).

2 Thompson, K.; Harris, M.; Benjamini, E.; Mitchell, G.; Noble, M.: Cellular and humoral immunity: a distinction in antigenic recognition. Nature new Biol. *238:* 20–21 (1972).

3 Ishizaka, K.; Kishimoto, T.; Delepasse, G.; King, T.P.: Immunogenic properties of modified antigen E. I. Response of specific determinants for T cells in denatured antigen and polypeptide chains. J. Immun. *113:* 70–77 (1974).

4 Schirrmacher, V.; Wigzell, H.: Immune responses against native and chemically modified albumins in mice. II. Effect of alternation of electric charge and conformation on the humoral antibody response and helper T cell responses. J. Immun. *113:* 1635–1643 (1974).

5 Watts, T.H.; Brian, A.A.; Kappler, J.W.; Marrack, P.; McConnell, H.M.: Antigen presentation by supported planar membranes containing affinity purified I-A^d. Proc. natn. Acad. Sci. USA *81:* 7564–7568 (1984).

6 Senyk, G.; Williams, E.B.; Nitecki, D.; Goodman, J.W.: The functional disection of an antigen molecule: specificity of humoral and cellular immune responses to glucagon. J. exp. Med. *133:* 1294–1308 (1971).

7 Maizels, R.M.; Clarke, J.A.; Harvey, M.A.; Miller, A.; Sercarz,. E.E.: Epitope specificity of the T cell proliferative response to lysozyme: proliferative T cells react predominantly to different determinants from those recognized by B cells. Eur. J. Immunol. *10:* 509–515 (1980).

8 Babbitt, B.P.; Allen, P.M.; Matsueda, G.; Haber, E.; Unanue, E.R.: Binding of immunogenic peptides to Ia histocompatibility molecules. Nature *317:* 359–361 (1985).

9 Buus, S.; Colon, S.; Smith, C.; Freed, J.M.; Miles, C.; Grey, H.M.: Interaction between a processed ovalbumin peptide and Ia molecules. Proc. natn. Acad. Sci. USA *83:* 3968–3971 (1986).

10 Godfrey, W.L.; Lewis, G.K.; Goodman, J.W.: The anatomy of an antigen molecule: functional subregion of *L*-tyrosine-*p*-azobenzenenarsonate. Mol. Immunol. *21:* 969–978 (1984).

11 Werdelin, O.: Chemically related antigens compete for presentation by accessory cells to T cell. J. Immun. *129:* 1883–1891 (1982).

12 Rock, K.I.; Benacerraf, B.: Inhibition of antigen-specific T lymphocyte activation by structurally related Ir gene-controlled polymers. Evidence of specific competition for accessory cell antigen presentation. J. exp. Med. *157:* 1618–1634 (1983).

13 Babbitt, B.; Matsueda, G.; Haber, E.; Unanue, E.R.; Allen, P.M.: Antigen competition at the level of peptide-Ia binding. Proc. natn. Acad. Sci. USA *83:* 4509–4513 (1986).

14 Guillet, J.G.; Lai, M.Z.; Briner, T.J.; Buus, S.; Sette, A.; Grey, H.M.; Smith, J.A.; Gefter, M.L.: Immunological self, nonself discrimination. Science *235:* 865–870 (1987).

15 Bjorkman, P.J.; Saper, M.A.; Samraoui, B.; Bennett, W.S.; Strominger, J.L.; Wiley, D.C.: The foreign antigen binding site and T cell recognition regions of class I histocompatibility antigens. Nature *329:* 512–518 (1987).

16 Brown, J.H.; Jardetzky, T.; Saper, M.A.; Samraoui, B., Bjorkman, P.J.; Wiley, D.C.: A hypothetical model of the foreign antigen binding site of class II histocompatibility molecules. Nature *329:* 845–850 (1988).

17 Goodman, J.W.; Sercarz, E.E.: The complexity of structures involved in T cell activation. Am. Rev. Immunol. *1:* 465–498 (1983).

18 Heber-Katz, E.; Hansburg, D.; Schwartz, R.H.: The Ia molecule of the antigen-presenting cell plays a critical role in immune response gene regulation of T cell activation. J. mol. cell. Immunol. *1:* 3–14 (1983).

19 Hertel-Wulff, B.; Goodman, J.W.; Fathman, C.G.; Lewis, G.K.: Arsonate-specific murine T cell clones. I. Genetic control and antigen specificity. J. exp. Med. *157:* 987–997 (1983).

20 Manca, F.; Clarke, J.A.; Miller, A.; Sercarz, E.E.; Shastri, N.: A limited region within hen egg-white lysozyme serves as the focus for a diversity of T cell clones. J. Immun. *133:* 2075–2078 (1984).

21 Cease, K.B.; Berkower, I.; York-Jolley, J.; Berzofsky, J.A.: T cell clones specific for an amphipathic alpha helical region of sperm whale myglobin show differing fine specificities for synthetic peptides: a multiview/single structure interpretation of immunodominance. J. exp. Med. *164:* 1779–1784 (1986).

22 Townsend, A.R.M.; Rothbard, J.B.; Gotch, F.M.; Bahadur, G.; Wraith, D.; McMichael, A.J.: The epitopes of influenza nucleoprotein recognized by cytotoxic T lymphocytes can be defined with short synthetic peptides. Cell *44:* 959–968 (1986).

23 Morrison, L.A.; Lukacher, A.E.; Braciale, V.L.; Fan, D.P.; Braciale, T.J.: Differences in antigen presentation to MHC class I- and class II-restricted influenza virus-specific cytolytic T lymphocyte clones. J. exp. Med. *163:* 903–921 (1986).

24 Kabat, E.A.: The nature of an antigenic determinant. J. Immun. *97:* 1–11 (1966).

25 Goodman, J.W.: Antigenic determinants and antibody combining sites; in Sela, The antigens, vol. III, pp. 127–187 (Academic Press, New York 1975).

26 Benjamin, D.C.; Berzofsky, J.A.; East, I.J.; Gurd, F.R.N.; Hannum, C.; Leach, S.J.; Margoliash, E.; Michael, J.G.; Miller, A.; Prager, E.M.; Reichlin, M.; Sercarz, E.E.; Smith-Gill, S.J.; Todd, P.A.; Wilson, A.C.: The antigenic structure of proteins: a reappraisal. A. Rev. Immunol. *2:* 67–101 (1984).

27 Schroer, J.A.; Bender, T.; Feldmann, R.J.; Kim, K.J.: Mapping epitopes on the insulin molecule using monoclonal antibodies. Eur. J. Immunol. *13:* 693–700 (1983).

28 Niman, H.L.; Houghten, R.A.; Walker, L.A.; Reisfeld, R.A.; Wilson, I.A.; Hogle, J.M.; Lerner, R.A.: Generation of protein-reactive antibodies by short peptides is an event of high frequency: implications for the sturctural basis of immune recognition. Proc. natn. Acad. Sci. USA *80:* 4949–4953 (1983).

29 Altschuh, D.; Al Moudallal, Z.; Briand, J.P.; Van Regenmortel, M.H.V.: Immunochemical studies of tobacco mosaic virus. VI. Attempts to localize viral epitopes with monoclonal antibodies. Mol. Immunol. *22:* 329–337 (1985).

30 Fieser, T.M.; Tainer, J.A.; Geysen, H.M.; Houghten, R.A.; Lerner, R.A.: Influence of protein flexibility and peptide conformation on reactivity of monoclonal anti-peptide antibodies with a protein α-helix. Proc. natn. Acad Sci. USA *84:* 8568–8572 (1987).

31 Moudallal, Al.Z.; Briand, J.P.; Van Regenmortel, M.H.V.: A major part of the polypeptide chain of tobacco mosaic virus protein is antigenic. EMBO J. *4:* 1231–1235 (1985).

32 Hansburg, D.; Fairwell, T.; Schwartz, R.H.; Appella, E.: The T lymphocyte response to cytochrome *c*. IV. Distinguishable sites on a peptide antigen which affect antigenic strength and memory. J. Immun. *131:* 319–324 (1983).

33 Hansburg, D.; Heber-Katz, E.; Fairwell, T.; Appella, E.: Major histocompatibility complex-controlled antigen presenting cell expressed-specificity of T cell antigen recognition. J. exp. Med. *158:* 25–39 (1983).

34 Pincus, M.R.; Gerewitz, F.; Schwartz, R.H.; Scheraga, H.A.: Correlation between the conformation of cytochrome *c* peptides and their stimulatory activity in a T lymphocyte proliferation assay. Proc. natn. Acad. Sci. USA *80:* 3297–3300 (1983).

35 Goodman, J.W.; Fong, S.; Lewis, G.K.; Kamin, R.; Nitecki, D.E.; Der Balian, G.: Antigen structure and lymphocyte activation. Immunol. Rev. *39:* 36–59 (1978).

36 Schlossman, S.: Antigen recognition: the specificity of T cell involved in the cellular immune response. Transplant. Rev. *10:* 97–111 (1972).

37 Thomas, D.W.; Hsieh, K.-H.; Schauster, J.L.; Wilner, G.D.: Fine specificity of genetic regulation of guinea pig T lymphocyte responses to angiotensin II and related peptides. J. exp. Med. *153:* 583–594 (1981).

38 Rothbard, J.B.; Taylor, W.R.: A sequence pattern common to T cell epitopes. EMBO J. *7:* 93–100 (1988).

39 Livingstone, A.M.; Fathman, C.G.: The structure of T cell epitopes. A. Rev. Immunol. *37:* 477–501 (1987).

40 Heber-Katz, E.; Valentine, S.; Dietzschold, B.; Burns-Purzycki, C.: Overlapping T cell antigenic sites on a synthetic peptide fragment from herpes simplex virus glycoprotein D, the degenerate MHC restriction elicited, and functional evidence for antigen-Ia interaction. J. exp. Med. *167:* 275–287 (1988).

41 Kronenberg, M.; Siu, G.; Hood, L.E.; Shastri, N.: The molecular genetics of the T cell antigen receptor and T cell antigen recognition. A. Rev. Immunol. *167:* 529–591 (1986).

42 Berzofsky, J.A.; Cease, K.B.; Cornette, J.L.; Spouge, J.L.; Margalit, H.; Berkower, I.J.; Good, M.F.; Miller, L.H.; Delisi, C.: Protein antigenic structures recognized by T cells: potential applications to vaccine design. Immunol. Rev. *98:* 9–52 (1987).

43 Shastri, N.; Oki, A.; Miller, A.; Sercarz, E.E.: Distinct recognition phenotypes exist for T cell clones specific for small peptide regions of proteins. Implications for the mechanisms underlying major histocompatibility complex-restricted antigen recognition and clonal deletion models of immune response gene defects. J. exp. Med. *162:* 332–345 (1985).

44 Suzuki, G.; Schwartz, R.H.: The pigeon cytochrome *c*-specific T cell response of low responder mice. I. Identification of antigenic determinants on fragment 1 to 65. J. Immun. *136:* 230–239 (1986).

45 Spragg, J.H.; Goodman, J.W.: Arsonate-specific murine T cell clones. IV. Properties of I-E- and I-A-restricted clones. J. Immun. *138:* 1169–1177 (1987).

46 Roy, S.; Gold, D.P.; Leskowitz, S.: ABA-specific responses are I region restricted by the carriers used for immunization. J. Immun. *136:* 3160–3165 (1986).

47 Regnier, D.; Seman, M.: Immune response to the *p*-azobenzenenarsonate (ABA)-GAT conjugate. II. Hapten-specific T cells induced with ABA-GAT in GAT responder X nonresponder F1 hybrids are restricted to the nonresponder halotype. J. Immun. *130:* 573–578 (1983).

48 Hedrick, S.M.; Matis, L.A.; Hecht, T.T.; Samelson, L.E.; Longo, D.L.; Heber-Katz, E.; Schwartz, R.H.: The fine specificity of antigen and Ia determinant recognition by T cell hybridoma clones specific for pigeon cytochrome *c*. Cell *30:* 141–152 (1982).

49 Mathis, D.J.; Benoist, C.O.; Williams, V.E.; Kanter, M.R.; McDevitt, H.O.: The murine Eα immune response gene. Cell *32:* 745–754 (1983).

50 Mengle-Gaw, L.; McDevitt, H.: Allelic variation in the murine Ia β-chain genes; in Sercarz, Cantor, Chess, Regulation of the immune system. UCLA Symp. on Molecular and Cellular Biology (new ser.), vol. 18, pp. 29–46 (Liss, New York 1984).

51 Allen, P.M.; Matsueda, G.R.; Evans, R.J.; Dunbar, J.B.; Marshall, G.R.; Unanue, E.R.: Identification of the T cell and Ia contact residues of a T cell antigenic epitope. Nature *327:* 713–715 (1987).

52 Sette, A.; Buus, S.; Colon, S.; Smith, J.A.; Miles, C.; Grey, H.M.: Structural characteristics of an antigen required for its interaction with Ia and recognition by T cells. Nature *328:* 395–399 (1987).

53 Unanue, E.R.: Antigen-presenting function of the macrophage. A. Rev. Immunol. *2:* 395–428 (1984).

54 Kabat, E.A.; Wei, T.T.; Reid-Miller, M.; Perry, H.M.; Gottesman, K.S.: Sequences of proteins of immunological interest; 4th ed., p. 373 (US Dept. of Health and Human Services, Washington 1987).

55 Norton, F.L.; Davis, C.B.; Jones, P.P; Goodman, J.W.: Presentation of arsonate-tyrosine to cloned T cells by L cells transfected with class II genes; in Schook, Tew,

Antigen-presenting cells: diversity, differentiation and regulation, pp. 193–199 (Liss, New York 1988).
56 Norton, F.L.; Davis, C.; Jones, P.; Goodman, J.W.: Manuscript in preparation.
57 Davis, C.; Norton, F.; Goodman, J.; Gammon, G.; Sercarz, E.; Mitchell, D.; Steinman, L.; Jones, P.: The role of polymorphic regions of the I-A molecule in antigen presentation. FASEB J. *2:* A671 (1988).
58 Good, M.F.; Maloy, W.L.; Lunde, M.N.; Margalit, H.; Cornette, J.L.; Smith, G.L.; Moss, B.; Miller, L.H.; Berzofsky, J.A.: Construction of synthetic immunogen: use of new T-helper epitope on malaria circumsporozoite protein. Science *235:* 1059–1062 (1987).
59 Good, M.F.; Pombo, D.; Maloy, W.L; Cruz, V.F. de la; Miller, L.H.; Berzofsky, J.A.: Parasite polymorphism present within minimal T cell epitopes of *Plasmodium falciparum* circumsporozoite protein. J. Immun. *140:* 1645–1650 (1988).
60 Klotz, F.W.; Hudson, D.E.; Coon, H.G.; Miller, L.H.: Vaccination-induced variation in the 140 kD merozoite surface antigen of *Plasmodium knowlesi* malaria. J. exp. Med. *165:* 359–367 (1987).
61 Milich, D.R.; Hughes, J.L.; McLachlan, A.; Thornton, G.B.; Moriarty, A.: Hepatitis B synthetic immunogen comprised of nucleocapsid T-cell sites and an envelope B-cell epitope. Proc. natn. Acad. Sci. USA *85:* 1610–1614 (1988).
62 Robey, W.G.; Arthur, L.O.; Matthews, T.J.; Langlois, A.; Copeland, T.D.; Lerche, N.W.; Oroszlan, S.; Bolognesi, D.P.; Gilden, R.V.; Fischinger, P.J.: Prospect for prevention of human immunodeficiency virus infection: purified 120-kDa envelope glycoprotein induces neutralizing antibody. Proc. natn. Acad. Sci. USA *83:* 7023–7027 (1986).
63 Fischinger, P.J.; Robey, W.G.; Koprowski, H.; Gallo, R.C.; Bolognesi, D.P.: Current status and strategies for vaccines against diseases induced by human T-cell lymphotropic retroviruses (HTLV-I, -II, -III). Cancer Res. *45:* 4694s–4699 (1985).
64 Cease, K.B.; Margalit, H.; Cornette, J.L.; Putney, S.D.; Robey, W.G.; Ouyang, C.; Streicher, H.Z.; Fischinger, P.J.; Gallo, R.C.; DeLisi, C.; Berzofsky, J.A.: Helper T-cell antigenic site identification in the acquired immunodeficiency syndrome virus gp120 envelope protein and induction of immunity in mice to the native protein using a 16-residue synthetic peptide. Proc. natn. Acad. Sci. USA *84:* 4249–4253 (1987).
65 Good, M.F.; Pombo, D.; Quakyi, I.A.; Riley, E.M.; Houghten, R.A.; Menon, A.; Alling, D.W.; Berzofsky, J.A.; Miller, L.H.: Human T-cell recognition of the circumsporozoite protein of *Plasmodium falciparum*: immunodominant T-cell domains map to the polymorphic regions of the molecule. Proc. natn. Acad. Sci. USA *85:* 1199–1203 (1988).
66 Brett, S.J.; Cease, K.B.; Berzofsky, J.A.: Influences of antigen processing on the expression of the T cell repertoire: evidence for MHC-specific hindering structures on the products of processing. J. exp. Med. *168:* 351–373 (1988).

Joel W. Goodman, PhD, Department of Microbiology and Immunology,
University of California, San Francisco, CA 94143 (USA)

Sercarz E (ed): Antigenic Determinants and Immune Regulation. Chem Immunol.
Basel, Karger, 1989, vol 46, pp 23–48

T Cell Clones and Monoclonal Antibodies: Immunologic Probes of Major Histocompatibility Complex Class I Molecules

Jeffrey A. Bluestone, Terry Potter

Ben May Institute, University of Chicago, Chicago, Ill., and Department of Pathology, Albert Einstein College of Medicine, Bronx, N.Y., USA

Introduction

In this review, we will focus on two major approaches designed to delineate the structure of the class I molecule involved in immune reactions in the murine and human systems. The first approach has been the use of in-vivo- and in-vitro-derived major histocompatibility complex (MHC) variants that express class I molecules with substitutions at one or a few amino acids. These mutants have been derived by immune selection or site-directed mutagenesis and have been useful in dissecting fine structural differences among MHC molecules. The second major approach has been the use of genetically engineered MHC genes. These novel hybrid MHC genes, referred to as exon shuffles, have been constructed using conserved nucleotide sequences in selected introns as sites for restriction enzyme digestion and religation. The hybrid genes are then expressed in cells after transfection and their product can be examined for the conservation of serological and T-cell-recognized determinants.

Although much information has been gained from these studies, the recent completion of the crystal structure of a human class I MHC molecule has provided a three-dimensional structural framework to integrate the functional data. The purpose of this chapter is to review our own and other functional data and assimilate the findings into our present understanding of the MHC structure, in an attempt to develop a unifying model to understand the influence of MHC class I structure on immune recognition.

Organization and Structure of MHC Class I Molecules

The murine MHC consists of between 23 and 27 relatively homologous class I genes located on chromosome 17 [1–4]. These genes can be divided into two groups: (1) The classical H-2 transplantation antigens, encoded by 3–8 genes located in 3 regions (*H-2K*, *H-2D*, and *H-2L*), which are found on the surface of virtually all cells and act as target antigens for cytotoxic cells and some helper T cells [5–9]. (2) The remaining class I genes are located telomeric to the *H-2L* region [10–11]. These genes, which have serologically localized to the regions, *Q* and *TL*, display much less polymorphism than the classical transplantation antigens, and are limited in their tissue distribution. The selective expression of some of these molecules on certain T cell subsets within the thymus suggests they may play a role in thymic development [12]. However in some cases these class I molecules can serve as target structures for alloreactive cytolytic T cells (CTL), although they have not been shown to function as restricting elements for antigen [13–15]. The molecules encoded by the MHC class I genes are 40,000–45,000 molecular weight glycoproteins that associate with β_2-microglobulin, a 12,000 molecular weight protein located on chromosome 2 [16, 17].

MHC class I genes are composed of 8 exons encoding a leader sequence, three external domains (α_1, α_2, and α_3) of approximately 90 residues each, a transmembrane portion (TM), and an intracytoplasmic carboxyl terminus (IC) [11]. Overall, the class I genes within a species are approximately 80–90% homologous. However, each gene within the species is highly polymorphic, so individual strains express a larger number of antigenically distinct class I proteins. The majority of the polymorphism found in the class I molecules is localized to the α_1 and α_2 domains. In fact, the immune system appears to focus on these polymorphic regions of the α_1 and α_2 domains, since T cells can readily distinguish individual class I molecules. Yet, although the α_3 domain of the class I gene is relatively conserved, all three external domains are considered integral in immune response gene control and MHC restriction [18–20].

Recently, a human class I molecule, HLA-A2, has been purified from papain digested plasma membranes and crystallized to determine its tertiary structure [21]. A schematic representation of the molecule is shown in figure 1. The three external domains (α_1, α_2, and α_3) and β_2-microglobulin form two pairs of structurally similar domains. The membrane-proximal α_3 and β_2-microglobulin segments each form immunoglobulin-like domains based on a β-sandwich structure composed of two anti-parallel β-pleated sheets. The α_3 and β_2-microglobulin domains intimately contact each other at the β-pleated sheets. In contrast, the α_1 and α_2 segments combine to form a single domain consisting of a floor, composed of a single β-pleated sheet, which is overlayed by two α helices (one encoded by the α_1 domain and the other the α_2 domain). A long, deep groove between the helices is evident in the three-dimensional structure. The sides of the groove are formed by the

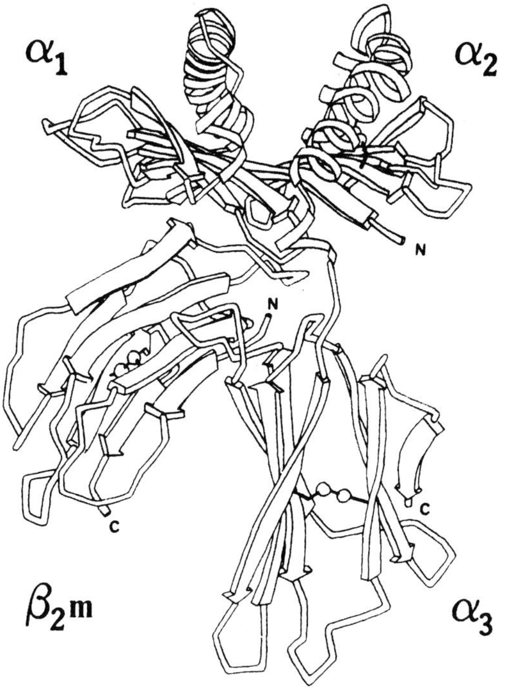

Fig. 1. Schematic representation of the HLA-A2 molecule. This figure has been reprinted by permission from Nature *329:* 506 (1987) ©, Macmillan Journals Limited.

side chains of the amino acids of the α helices and the base formed by the β-pleated sheet α_1/α_2 domain.

Interestingly, an electron density, unaccounted for by any segment of the HLA molecule, was found within the α_1/α_2 groove in the native crystal structure. It is generally accepted that T lymphocytes recognize antigens in the context of molecules encoded by genes in the MHC [22–25]. MHC class-II-restricted T cells usually recognize processed rather than native forms of antigen on the surface of class-II-bearing antigen-presenting cells [26–28]. It has recently been shown that short synthetic peptides corresponding to the antigenic sites of the influenza nucleoprotein (NP) can render uninfected target cells susceptible to lysis by NP-specific class-I-restricted CTL. This suggests that class-I-restricted recognition might also involve processed antigenic fragments [29]. This model applies generally to antigens normally expressed as integral membrane proteins at the cell surface, and is consistent with the notion that peptides can bind MHC class I molecules directly, and suggest that electron density within the α_1/α_2

groove could represent a processed peptide bound to the HLA molecule [91].

It should be emphasized that this three-dimensional structure is of a single MHC class I molecule and polymorphisms among the class I proteins may substantially alter the tertiary conformation. However, as will be seen later, the structure of other class I molecules can be modeled on the HLA-A2 structure [30]. In fact, recent studies suggest that class II molecules may also be modeled on the same structure [31]. Thus, for the first time functional information gained from serological and T cell reactivity studies can be assessed in the context of this three-dimensional structure. We will examine the functional effects of altering class I molecules within the realm of possible changes of the tertiary crystallographic structure.

Studies Examining α_1/α_2 Integrity in Immune Recognition

As mentioned earlier, one broad approach to determining the roles of individual regions of a class I molecule in antibody and T cell recognition has been the use of genetically manipulated class I genes. Initial studies showed that cDNA and genomic clones of class I genes could be introduced into mouse L cells and detected as protein on the cell surface by mAbs. Further studies showed that these gene products could be recognized by alloreactive and MHC-restricted antigen-specific CTL, providing the basis for an analysis of the need for molecular integrity of the MHC molecule in immunorecognition [32–35].

Therefore, hybrid MHC genes, constructed from different class I genes, were transfected into cells and examined for T cell and mAb recognition [36–53]. For example, the exons encoding the α_1/α_2 domain of the K^b gene was spliced to the exons encoding the α_3, TM, and IC domains of the D^b gene [36]. Results of some of these studies are summarized in table 1. Serologic analysis of these transfectants showed that the binding of most mAbs could be mapped to one of the two external domains (α_1/α_2). Extensive serology has been performed on the exon shuffled MHC class I molecules. Allen et al. [36] and Bluestone et al. [47] examined monoclonal antibody binding to exon-shuffled $H\text{-}2K^b$ and $H\text{-}2D^b$ genes between the α_1/α_2 and α_3 encoding exons so that the domain shuffled molecules expressed on transfected L cells consisted of $K^b/K^b/D^b$ or $D^b/D^b/K^d$ (referring to the origin of the $\alpha_1/\alpha_2/\alpha_3$ domains). Most mAb specific for K^b or D^b molecule reacted with the α_1 and/or α_2 domains although the mAb, 28–14–8, reacted with the α_3 domain of H-2D^b. Similar results have been observed in other haplotypes as well (i.e. $L^d/L^d/D^d$, $K^k/K^k/K^d$ and

Table 1. Summary of CTL recognition of MHC class I recombinant gene products

Recombinant gene			Alloreactive CTL recognition		Self MHC + X recognition
α_1	α_2	α_3/TM/IC	bulk	clones	
K^b	K^b	D^d	+	+	+(FLU)
K^b	D^b	D^b	−	−	−(FLU)
D^b	K^b	K^b	−	−	−(FLU)
K^d	K^d	K^k	+	+	+(FLU)
K^d	K^k	K^k	−	2% (5:41)	−(FLU)
K^k	K^d	K^d	−	12% (6:30)	−(FLU)
D^d	Q7	D^d	−	NT	−(VSV)
D^d	L^d	L^d	+	44% (7:16)	+(FLU)
D^d	D^d/L^d	L^d	+/−	−	−(VSV)
L^d	D^d	D^d	−	−	−(VSV)

NT = Not tested.

Qa/L^d). In these studies, the reactivity of all T cells, both alloreactive and antigen-specific, depended on the origin of the α_1/α_2 domain.

Once it became clear that the majority, if not all, conventional CTL recognize polymorphisms dependent on amino acids resident in the α_1 and α_2 domains, attempts were made to delineate independently the role of the α_1 and α_2 domains in antibody and T cell recognition. A variety of laboratories have studied the immune recognition of mouse fibroblasts transfected with hybrid MHC gene products including exon shuffles between nonhomologous α_1 and α_2 exons of D^d/L^d, L^d/D^d, K^b/D^b, D^b/K^b, K^k/K^d, K^d/K^k and Qa/L^d (referring to the origin of the $\alpha_1/\alpha_2\alpha_3$ domains) [37, 38, 41, 42, 45, 47, 48]. Most mAb have been provisionally mapped to the α_1 or α_2 encoded protein structures. However, in many instances, the mAb have weak binding to the hybrid MHC molecules [47] and may interact with a site controlled by both the α_1 and α_2 domains. In addition, a few mAb, which have been previously mapped to the α_1 or α_2 domain in a certain hybrid molecule, do not react with the same domain when shuffled with exons from other haplotypes suggesting that these particular epitopes may be indirectly controlled by another domain [48].

Hybrid MHC recognition by alloreactive and MHC-restricted antigen-specific T cells was significantly less well preserved. Both in bulk culture and limiting dilution analysis, the CTL activity on α_1/α_2 exon shuffled gene products was drastically reduced (table 1). These results are consistent with the three-dimensional structure of the α_1/α_2 domain in that, unlike mAbs, it would appear that recognition of MHC class I molecules

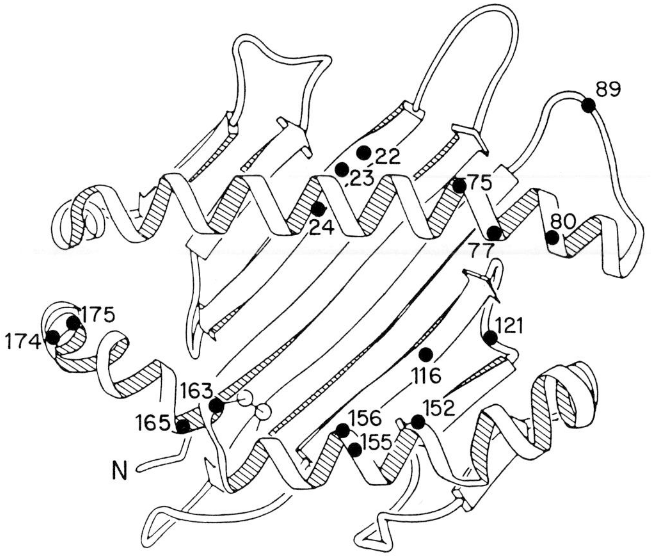

Fig. 2. Location of the altered amino acid residues of in vivo H-2K^{bm} mutants on a schematic representation of the H-2K^{b} model structure. The K^{b} model depicts the α_1 and α_2 domain portion of the K^{b} molecule. The amino-terminal is indicated by 'N', the β-strands by flat arrow ribbons, and the α helices by coiled ribbons. Residues 1–90 form the α_1 domain which is comprised of the first four β strands from the amino-terminal, and the α_1 helix (residues 58–84). The α_2 domain consists of residues 91–182, and is formed by the four β strands (immediately following the α_1 helix), and the two α_2 helices (residues 138–180). The positions of the amino acid substitutions are identified by numbers. This figure, as well as figure 3, has been adapted from Bjorkman et al. [21] and Ajitkumar et al. [30].

by T cells is dependent on the intimate contact of the α_1 and α_2 helical regions which create the peptide groove (fig. 2).

It should be noted that one hybrid MHC molecule can be recognized efficiently by alloreactive and antigen-specific CTL [42]. Cells expressing the $D^d_{\alpha1}/L^d_{\alpha2}$ hybrid molecule were lysed by H-2D^d-, H-2L^d- and influenza-specific CTL. In contrast, the reciprocal exon shuffle, $L^d_{\alpha1}/D^d_{\alpha2}$ was not recognized [48]. Interestingly, a mouse strain B10.D2-H-2^{dm1} (dm1) is an in-vivo-derived *H-2D^d/L^d* exon shuffle resulting from the fusion of the *H-2D^d* and *H-2L^d* genes. The fusion occurred between residues 122 and 155 resulting in the α_1 and most of the α_2 domain derived from H-2D^d while the C-terminal amino acids of the α_2 domain are H-2L^d [54]. Studies have shown that both anti-H-2D^d and anti-H-2L^d-specific CTL cross-react on dm1 target cells, consistent with the studies of the H-2D^d/L^d exon shuffle which retained alloreactive determinants characteristic of both parents [55].

Similar results have been found with a naturally occurring human domain-shuffled molecule where EBV/HLA-A2-specific CTL can recognize target cells expressing the HLA-Aw69 molecule which expresses *HLA-Aw68* sequences in the α_1 and *HLA-A2*-sequences in the α_2 domains [56, 57].

The reason that T cell recognition is preserved on certain hybrid molecules is not clear. In the case of the $D^d_{\alpha 1}/L^d_{\alpha 2}$-encoded hybrid molecule there are fewer changes in the α_2 domain between H-2L^d and H-2D^d (11 amino acid residues) compared with some other allelic pairs (i.e. 16–17 residues). However, where the changes are located may be more critical than the number of changes. For instance, several of the amino acid changes between H-2L^d and H-2D^d are localized to amino acids in the α-helical turns which face away from the peptide groove and would not be predicted to have any effect on CTL recognition.

Recent studies have utilized more sophisticated molecular approaches to molecularly alter segments of class I molecules. Intradomain exon shuffles have been derived and examined for both serological and T cell recognition. Scholler et al. [58] generated hybrid genes among the H-2K^d, K^k and K^b molecules within the α_2 domain such that they differ from wild type α_1/α_2 only at the COOH-terminus of the domain, like the *dm1* mutant (amino acids 142–182). In contrast to a complete α_1/α_2 exon-shuffle of the H-2K^k and H-2K^d MHC molecule, which destroyed all alloreactive and virus-specific cytolytic activity, the partial exon shuffle retained the majority of the target activity. Further studies were performed by Abastado et al. [59] in which intradomain recombinants between *H-2K^d* and *D^d* were produced using a technique based on in vivo gene recombination in *E. coli.* These intradomain shuffled genes have allowed for the fine mapping of serological epitopes on the MHC class I molecules. In addition, the specificity of presentation of two HLA peptides was linked to two distinct regions within the α_2 domain of K^d indicating that the recognition of certain antigens can be mapped using these chimeric molecules. However, our findings suggested that alloreactive CTL activity remained intact only when the majority of the α_1/α_2 domains were homologous in origin.

Role of Individual Amino Acids within the α_1 and α_2 Domains of Class I Molecules in T Cell Recognition

Initial studies of the effects of individual amino acids on T cell recognition focused on the use of in-vivo-derived spontaneous MHC class I mutants, which differed from the wild-type molecule by one or a limited number of amino acids [60–92]. The most widely studied of these systems is the *bm* series of *H-2K^b* mutants, originally detected by reciprocal skin

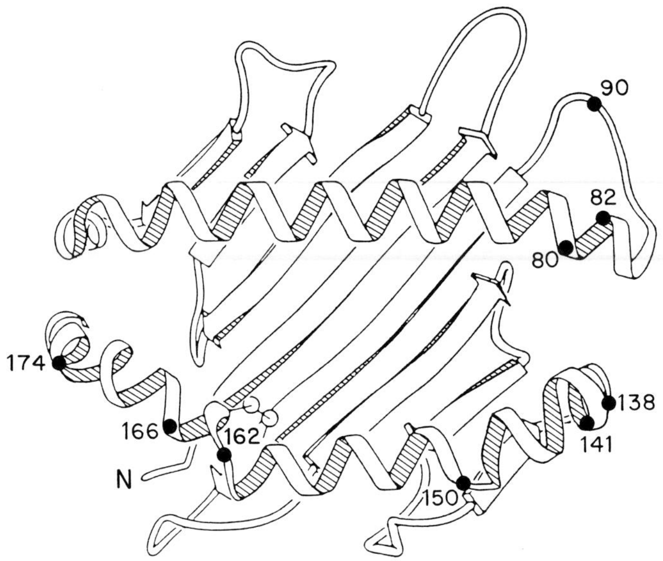

Fig. 3. Location of the altered amino acid residues of in-vitro-derived H-2K^{bm} mutants on a schematic representation of the H-2K^{b} model structure. The K^{b} molecule is depicted as in figure 2.

graft rejection [62–64]. Amino acid and/or nucleotide sequencing revealed that all of these mutations have occurred within the α_1 or α_2 domains [65] and appear to be the consequence of gene conversion-like events resulting from the insertion of DNA from other class I molecules into the wild type K^b gene [83, 84]. Recently, the H-2K^{b} three-dimensional structure has been generated based on the HLA-A2 model structure [30] (fig. 3). This H-2K^{b} model provides the basis for determining the location of individual amino acid changes in the mutants. For the most part, the amino acid changes appear to be localized to the α helical regions of the MHC molecule (i.e. amino acid 70–90 and 150–175; fig. 3, table 2) although in one strain, bm8, the changes are localized to the β-sheet base of the peptide groove.

Whereas structural differences among the H-2K^{b} molecules of these wild type and mutant mice can be readily distinguished by alloreactive and foreign-peptide-specific self-restricted CTL and by skin grafting [66–78], the mutant mice are rarely distinguished using serological reagents [87–90]. In fact, the limited effects on antibody recognition of the in vivo derived mutants appear to predominantly affect epitopes encoded within the same domain (intradomain). These results had suggested that the α_1 and α_2 domains are unique entities within the molecule. In contrast, the extensive changes in T cell recognition appear to be localized to both the α_1 and α_2

Table 2. Amino acid alterations in in-vivo- and in-vitro-derived H-2K^b mutants

Mutants	Domain with mutation	Position of mutation	Amino acid change
In vitro			
R8.125	α_1	90	Gly to Asp
R8.24	α_1	80	Thr to Ile
R8.246	α_1	80	Thr to Ile
R8.208	α_1	82	Leu to Pro
R8.313	α_1	82	Leu to Phe
R8.127	α_2	138	Met to Lys
R8.14	α_2	141	Leu to Arg
R8.331	α_2	150	Ala to Pro
R8.341	α_2	162	Gly to Asp
R8.10	α_2	167	Trp to Arg
R8.347	α_2	166	Glu to Lys
In vivo			
bm3	α_1	77, 89	Asp to Ser Lys to Ala
bm19	α_1	80	Thr to Asn Asp to Ser
bm11	α_1	77, 80	Asp to Ser Thr to Asn
bm6	α_2	116, 121	Thr to Phe Cys to Arg
bm10	α_2	163, 165 174, 175	Thr to Ala Val to Met Lys to Glu Asn to Leu

domains (interdomain) as would be predicted by the three-dimensional structure of the MHC [91]. For example, the H-2K^b α_1-domain mutant bm3 (amino acids 77, 89) expresses serological changes in common with other mutants altered at a similar site within the α_1-domain (i.e. bm19, amino acid 80; and bm23, amino acid 75, 77) but not mutants altered in the α_2 domain (i.e. bm10, amino acids 163, 165, 174, 175 and bm1, amino acids 152, 155, 156). In contrast, the reactivity of a H-2K^b-specific CTL generated by an α_2 domain mutant mouse, K^{bm10}, was markedly reduced when examined on α_1-domain mutants such as bm3 or bm8 (amino acids 22, 23, 24). Thus, these studies predicted that the recognition of class I molecules is dependent on the interaction of the α_1 and α_2 domains. This supports the notion that T cell recognition of class I antigens is dependent on an interaction of the α_1 and α_2 domains, while antibodies may recognize different epitopes than T cells on the class I molecules and may be less influenced by the α_1/α_2 interaction.

However, since the bm mutants were identified by reciprocal skin graft rejection, specific amino acid changes in critical T-cell-dependent diversity regions of the MHC molecule may have been selected for. Therefore, a refinement has been to examine MHC molecules with single amino acid changes which were generated by mutagenesis of in vitro tumor lines [92–94]. These mutants, which were identified by the loss of specific serologically defined determinants, are useful since they have not been selected on the basis of T cell recognition. Somatic variants of K^b molecule were derived by negatively selecting chemically mutagenized, serologically altered tumor cells with a monoclonal anti-H-$2K^b$ antibody and positively selecting for H-$2K^b$ expressing cells [92].

For the most part, a detailed analysis of these mutants yielded similar results to the in vivo mutants [30, 92, 95]. First, amino acid analysis of the in-vitro-selected mutants showed that all the changes were localized to polymorphic regions of the α_1 and α_2 domain, specifically in the α-helical regions (fig. 3b). MAb analyses of the mutants confirmed that the majority of serological epitopes were confined to spatially discrete, individual domains. In contrast, single amino acid changes at certain positions had profound effects on T cell recognition involving both the α_1 and α_2 domains. For instance, a single change at amino acid 174 (R8.353) eliminated the majority of reactivity of bulk alloreactive K^b-specific T cells. Similarly, changes at amino acid 82 (R8.313, ref. 96; R8.208) abolished the reactivity of the majority of bm8, bm11, bm10 anti-K^b-specific CTL.

Ajitkumar et al. [30] have noted that the influence of the mutation on T cell reactivity is based in part on their location and side chain orientation. The majority of amino acid residues that altered CTL recognition were located on the face of the α-helical structures that form the peptide groove suggesting that the T cell receptor reacts with both α-helical sequences and changes in this surface alter the ability of the T cell receptor to interact with the MHC molecule.

In addition, other residues including those altered in the *bm8* mutant (amino acids 22, 23, 24), which are located outside the α helices but within the peptide groove, also influence T cell recognition. These changes may alter the binding of foreign peptides to the class I molecule thus affecting T cell recognition. In view of this possibility, it has been hypothesized that at least some alloreactive T cells recognize foreign or self peptides in the context of the allogeneic MHC antigen. This hypothesis is supported by the recent studies of several investigators which suggested an involvement of tissue-specific self peptides in allorecognition. In these studies, CTL generated against human class I molecules expressed in transfected murine tumor lines recognized the allogeneic class I molecule in a H-2-restricted fashion.

Thus, conformational changes in α_1/α_2 can alter the accessibility of particular residues and therefore exert profound effects on determinants recognized by antibodies and T cells. In addition, such changes can influence T cell recognition by their effect on the binding of particular peptides.

Studies Analyzing Epitope Gains in Mutant and Hybrid MHC Class I Gene Products

The spontaneous in-vivo-derived H-2K^b mutants have both lost and gained allodeterminants on the K^b molecule [67, 70, 76, 86]. The new determinants have been shown to be most likely due to conformational alterations in the molecule which results in the creation of new epitopes on the MHC antigen. In fact, previous studies have suggested that a loss of allodeterminants is generally accompanied by a gain of new determinants [69]. However, such studies were carried out using in-vivo-derived mutants that were selected by the ability of mice expressing the wild type gene to reject grafts of the variants. Such a selection process may result in the isolation of only those mutations which result in profound alteration of the K^b molecule. Therefore, it was not surprising that the K^{bm} mice expressed novel determinants recognized by CTL. In addition, recent studies of the genes encoding the K^{bm} proteins have shown multiple nucleotide changes resulting in several amino acid changes in most of the mutants [65]. Therefore, the question as to the relationship between single amino acid changes and their effects on T cell recognition remained unanswered.

The in-vitro-derived H-2K^b variants provided an excellent model to study the effect of a single amino acid change on T cell recognition. In addition, since the variants were selected only for the loss of a single serologically defined determinant, no bias would exist toward alteration of sites specific to T cell recognition as compared to antibody recognition. We have shown that CTL can recognize novel determinants on two in vitro mutants, R8.24 and R8.246 [86]. It appears that the single amino acid change in R8.24 and R8.246 results in the creation of at least two new epitopes. One is shared with the bm6 and the other is a determinant shared with the bm3, bm11, bm19 and bm23 H-2K^b mutant molecules. As stated in table 1, the R8.24 and R8.246 mutants have been determined to be altered at amino acid 80 (thr $\rightarrow$ ile), which is located near the site of mutation in the bm3, bm11, bm19 and bm23 K^b mutant molecules (table 1). On the other hand, the H-2K^{bm6} molecule has been shown to have altered two amino acid residues in the α_2 domain (116 and 121). Thus, it would appear that there is an epitope created by the 116 and 121 change similar to that created by the amino acid change at position 80.

Examination of the three-dimensional structure does not provide insight into this finding (fig. 3). Although the amino acid changes in the bm6 and R8.24 mutants are close, the α carbon positions are still at least 10 Å apart. It, therefore, seems unlikely that these independent changes would result in similar epitopes.

Perhaps most striking, only these two of a total of 19 in-vitro-derived K^b mutants examined express novel determinants which could be detected by cytotoxic T cells. It is not yet clear why only these two mutants and no others have shown evidence of a gain of novel determinants. It is unlikely that the location of the mutation is responsible for the effect since other R8 variants which have alterations in the region of amino acids 80–90 (e.g. R8.313 amino acid 82 [leu → phe] [96]) do not reveal novel determinants. However, the present findings can now be placed in the context of the three-dimensional structure of the MHC class I molecule based on the X-ray crystallographic studies of Bjorkman et al. [21, 91] (fig. 3). Among all of the in vitro mutants analyzed, only the R8.24 and R8.246 mutants had alterations in amino acid side chains directed towards the antigen-binding site [30]. This might explain the finding that only these mutants create novel CTL recognizing alloantigens. For instance, this mutation might alter self peptide binding or alter the antigen-binding cleft and create epitopes which are recognized as allogeneic by T cells. Other mutations may affect T cell receptor binding sites but not create novel epitopes.

In this regard, recent findings from our laboratory and others suggest that changes in the MHC structure can significantly alter wild type epitopes without the concomitant gain in novel epitopes [47, 86, 97, 98]. Specifically, hybrid MHC molecules resulting from an exchange of α_1 domains between different genes results in most instances in the loss of all CTL recognition with little evidence for a gain in new determinants. Although some CTL can be generated in some experiments [47, 97, 98], limiting dilution analyses suggested at least a 100-fold difference in the precursor frequency of CTL specific for wild type versus exon-shuffled gene products.

Finally, site-directed mutagenesis has been used to localize critical amino acid residues in antibody and T cell binding determinants. Based on the prediction that amino acids 63–73 of the H-2D^d molecule were critical for allorecognition, selected amino acids within the H-2L^d molecule were changed from L → D and reexamined [99]. The results of these studies suggested that amino acid residues within this region controlled both serological and T cell epitopes. Thus, it would appear, as predicted by the three-dimensional structure of the MHC class I molecule, that the integrity of the α_1/α_2 domain is critical for T cell recognition although substitutions in selected regions can mimic or conserve/create selected sites for both mAb and CTL recognition.

Evidence for the Involvement of Determinants in the α_3 Domain in CTL Recognition

Exon Shuffling Experiments

As stated above, initial experiments which created hybrid genes by exon shuffling between murine *H-2D*^{d} and *H-2L*^{d} [18], *H-2K*^{b} and *H-2D*^{b} [36], and *H-2K*^{b}, *H-2K*^{d} and *H-2K*^{k} genes [41] demonstrated convincingly that class I reactive CTL recognizes determinants which reside in the α_1 and α_2, but not the α_3 domains. Analysis of hybrid genes constructed between the human *HLA-A2* and murine *H-2K*^{b} genes, however showed that substitution of the *H-2K*^{b} α_3 exon with the corresponding region from the *HLA-A2* gene reduced the reactivity with anti H-2K^b CTL [100]. Similarly replacement of the *HLA-A2* α_3 exon with the *H-2K*^{b} α_3 exon reduced the reactivity with anti HLA-A2 CTL. These findings raised the possibility that the α_3 domain did express determinants which were recognized by CTL. Analysis of the affinity and lytic ability of individual anti H-2K^b CTL clones for cells expressing the product of these hybrid genes suggested, however, that the reduced or complete loss of lysis by certain CTL clones was due to a conformation effect on the α_1/α_2 determinants by the replacement of the α_3 domain or failure of CD8 binding to the xenogeneic α_3 domain [101].

While the studies involving exon shuffling failed to identify a direct role for the α_3 domain in CTL recognition, they do not preclude the possibility that in addition to the allele specific polymorphic determinants residing in the α_1 and α_2 domains, there are conserved determinants on the class I molecule. A conserved determinant present on all class I molecules would have been maintained during the construction of hybrid genes and therefore would not have been identified in these studies. McCluskey et al. [102] constructed *H-2D*^{d} and *H-2L*^{d} genes in which exons encoding the α_1 and α_2 domains were deleted. While these truncated molecules were expressed on the cell surface as determined by reactivity with a mAb to the α_3 domain, CTL raised against the intact H-2D^d or H-2L^d molecule did not lyse cells expressing the truncated molecule. However, these truncated molecules could, upon in vivo priming and in vitro restimulation, elicit CTL that reacted with cells expressing the appropriate truncated molecule. Although the CTL were able to recognize the truncated gene products, these CTL were unable to recognize the intact MHC molecule expressing the homologous α_3 domain. The conclusion of these studies was that the α_3 domain expresses polymorphic determinants which can be recognized by T cells. However, it is possible that in the intact molecule these determinants are masked by the α_1 and α_2 domains. Alternatively, the CTL recognized the α_3 domain epitopes in an MHC restricted fashion via the self (H-2^k) molecule or the CTL may have recognized minor antigens expressed in the context of the truncated MHC gene products.

Inhibition of T Cell Reactivity by Antibodies to the α_3 Domain

An indication that determinants in the α_3 domain were recognized by CTL came from the observation that α_3 domain specific mAb could inhibit the reactivity of CTL [18, 103]. In the most comprehensive of these studies [1] it was clearly demonstrated that α_3 domain antibodies to H-2L^d (28–14–8) or H-2D^d (34–2–12) were as potent inhibitors of CTL reactivity as α_1/α_2 antibodies. Although these α_3 domain antibodies do not inhibit the binding of α_1/α_2 antibodies [104, and unpublished observations] it was possible that the effect of the α_3 antibodies on CTL was due to steric hindrance of the T cell receptor by the bound antibody. More recently, Connally et al. [105] have extended these observations and suggested that the inhibition of CTL reactivity by α_3 antibodies is in fact due to the blocking of recognition rather than steric hindrance. In these studies it was observed that the H-2L^d α_3 domain antibody (28–14–8) inhibited anti-H-2L^d CTL generated in a primary in vitro response, but not secondary CTL that were derived from spleen cells of mice primed in vivo with an H-2L^d incompatible skin graft. Furthermore, the addition of 28–14–8 to the in vitro culture inhibited the generation of primary, but not secondary, CTL. The reactivity of secondary CTL generated in the presence of 28–14–8 was not inhibited by the addition of anti-Lyt-2 antibody. These findings suggest that antibodies to the α_3 domain inhibit the reactivity of Lyt-2-dependent, but not Lyt-2-independent, CTL and raise the possibility that the Lyt-2 molecule recognizes some of the same residues as the α_3 domain antibodies.

Characterization of Mutations in the α_3 Domain

We have opted to study the role of the α_3 domain in recognition by T cells by isolation of somatic cell mutants through antibody mediated immunoselection. Cells expressing a mutant H-2L^d molecule that no longer reacted with the α_3 antibody (28–14–8), but did react with α_1/α_2 H-2L^d antibodies, were readily killed by anti H-2L^d CTL [106]. Although these mutations in the H-2L^d α_3 domain had no effect on the determinants recognized by anti-H-2L^d CTL, mutations in the α_3 domain of H-2D^d had profound effects on recognition by anti-H-2D^d CTL. In particular one cell line (ACCb34.2.12r4b$^-$), did not express the determinant recognized by the H-2D^d α_3 domain antibody 34–2–12. However, it still expressed the α_1/α_2 H-2D^d serological epitopes but was not killed by anti-H-2D^d alloreactive and antigen-specific CTL [107]. The nucleotide sequence of the mutant *H-2D^d* α_3 exon contains a single point mutation (guanosine to adenosine) at residue 227 that results in a lysine for glutamic acid substitution in the mutant molecule [108]. This alteration (determined by nucleotide sequencing) was consistent with the more basic nature of the mutant H-2D^d molecule as analyzed by isoelectric focusing/SDS polyacrylamide gel electrophesis. A comparison of the amino acid sequences of different MHC class I molecules reveals that the α_3 domain is much more conserved than the α_1/α_2 region. For example, H-2L^d and H-2D^d are identical from residue 200 to 260 with the exception of residue 227 (H-2D^d glutamic acid, H-2L^d aspartic acid) which our data suggests is required for the H-2D^d unique specificity recognized by the 34–2–12 antibody. Residue 227 is a conserved acidic group (either aspartic acid or glutamic acid) in all class I molecules. When this mutant gene was reproduced by oligonucleotide directed mutagenesis of a cloned *H-2D^d* gene and was transfected into various fibroblast and pre-B cell lines, identical phenotypic effects were observed. That is the gene product did not bind the 34–2–12 antibody and was not recognized by anti-H-2D^d CTL populations generated in primary in vitro responses. The lack of reactivity with CTL was not due to a substantial conformational effect of the substitution on α_1/α_2 epitopes, as the mutant H-2D^d molecule stimulated IL-2 production by the anti-H-2D^d reactive T cell hybridoma 3DT52.5.8.

To investigate whether the acid to base substitution had the same effect on CTL recognition in other class I molecules, we constructed hybrid genes consisting of the α_1 and α_2 exons of *H-2K^b* gene together with the α_3 exon of the wild type or mutant *H-2D^d* gene. Cells expressing H-2K^b α_1/α_2 in association with the wild type H-2D^d α_3 domain were readily killed by anti-H-2K^b CTL generated in a primary in vitro response. In contrast, cells expressing the hybrid gene containing the mutant H-2D^d α_3 domain were not killed by these primary CTL populations [109]. Therefore, the effect of the substitution on CTL recognition was not unique to H-2D^d as was apparent in other class I molecules. It should be noted that the HLA-A2 molecule has an aspartic acid corresponding to residue 227. Thus, other differences in the α_3 domain may also influence T cell recognition.

Possible Identification of the Receptor of the Conserved Determinant

To reconcile our observations on the effect of a point mutation in the α_3 domain of H-2D^d in the abrogation of recognition by T cells versus the exon shuffling experiments, we investigated the concept that there is a conserved determinant on murine class I molecules, dependent on amino acid residue 227, that is necessary for recognition by the CTL populations but not required for the reactivity of the IL-2-secreting hybridoma 3DT52.5.8. It should be noted that a determinant that is conserved, or identical, in all class I molecules would not have been identified in the exon shuffling experiments as such a determinant would have been preserved in the reconstructed hybrid genes. The exon shuffling experiments were specifically designed to examine only polymorphic determinants.

If there is a conserved determinant on MHC class I molecules then what is the receptor molecule on the T cell for this determinant? It seems probable that a receptor for a conserved determinant would not be as variable a molecule as the TCR$\alpha\beta$ complex. A likely candidate for this receptor is the Lyt-2 (CD8) molecule since antibody to the CD8 molecule generally inhibits class I reactive T cells [110, 111]. In addition, it has recently been demonstrated that it is necessary to transfect and express the CD8 gene, as well as TCR$\alpha\beta$ genes, in order to confer reactivity with class I molecules in recipient T cells [112, 113]. Although antibody to CD8 inhibits the reactivity of most class-I-reactive T cells (termed CD8-dependent), there are some CTL which are not inhibited by antibody to CD8 (termed CD8-independent) [114]. Such CD8-independent T cells are found in populations generated in in vitro secondary responses from the spleen cells of mice primed in vivo.

If CD8 is the receptor for the conserved determinant on the class I molecule and this determinant is destroyed in the mutant H-$2D^d$ molecule, then the effect of the mutation should be confined to the reactivity with CD8-dependent T cells whereas reactivity with CD8-independent cells should be unaffected. This suggestion was supported by the finding that the $CD8^-$ (and thus CD8-independent) T cell hybridoma 3DT52.5.8 recognized the mutant H-$2D^d$ molecule [108]. To further investigate this possibility we generated anti-H-$2K^b$ CTL in the presence of anti-CD8 antibody, resulting in CTL which were less susceptible to inhibition by antibody to CD8. Such CTL populations were cytotoxic for cells expressing the mutant α_3 H-$2D^d$ domain in association with the H-$2K^b$ α_1/α_2 domains [109]. Therefore although substitution of glutamic acid with lysine at residue 227 abrogates recognition by CD8-dependent CTL, it does not affect the reactivity with CD8-independent CTL. Our interpretation of these findings is that residue 227 contributes to a determinant on H-2 class I molecules that is recognized by the CD8 molecule on CTL and that the substitution at this residue destroys this determinant.

These results can once again be considered in the context of the three-dimensional structure of an HLA class I molecule (fig. 4). In this structure, residue 227 is located on the surface of the molecule, is solvent-accessible, and is at least 50 Å away from the α_1/α_2 peptide binding cleft [21; Saper and Wiley, personal communication]. The interface area for an antigen-antibody complex is approximately 30 by 20 Å (600 $Å^2$) and the T cell receptor α_1/α_2 class I molecule interface may encompass a slightly larger area of 39 by 20 Å (780 $Å^2$) [115, 116]. To encompass the area around residue 227 in addition to the α_1/α_2 helices the interface with the T cell receptor would have to be greater than these estimates. In contrast, if this region of the α_3 domain forms the determinant recognized by CD8, then CD8 and the TCR$\alpha\beta$ complex may bind to distinct regions of the class I

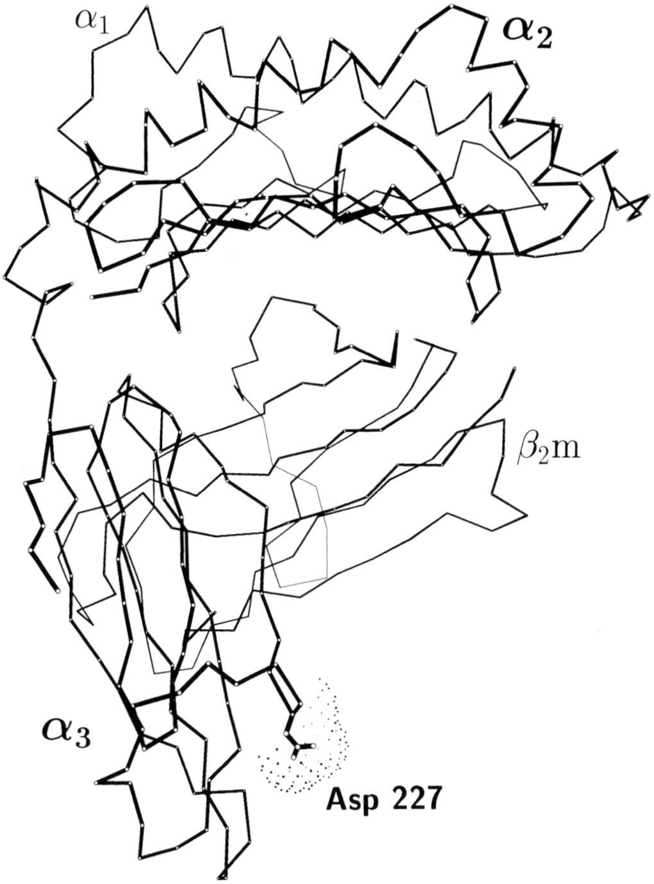

Fig. 4. Cα-backbone of HLA-A2 indicating the location of Asp 227 (Glu in H-2D[d]) on the surface of the α_3 domain approximately 50 Å from the antigen presentation site at the top of the molecule. The dots represent the water accessible surface surrounding the side chain. As suggested by line thickness, the α_2 and α_3 are closer to the viewer, α_1 and β_2-microglobulin are towards the rear. The figure was prepared by M.A. Saper and D.C. Wiley (Harvard University) using a program by D. Freymann and T.A. Jones.

molecule and not compete with each other for binding to particular common residues.

Summary and Implications

Although a great deal has been learned from studies such as those presented in this review, two major questions concerning T cell recognition of foreign antigen remain. First, what do the antigen-specific and alloreactive T cells recognize on the MHC molecule? Second, do certain accessory molecules recognize conserved determinants on the MHC class I molecule?

The studies summarized in this review would suggest that antigen-specific T cells recognize both the MHC molecule and a processed peptide that is physically bound to the antigen cleft created by the interaction of the α_1/α_2 α-helical sequence and the β-pleated sheet. During antigen-recognition the TCR complex interacts simultaneously with amino acid residues located in the α_1-encoded and the α_2-encoded helices as well as residues of the foreign peptide not involved in MHC binding. Changes in amino acids located within either α-helical sequence (especially those that have side chains directed upwards or into the antigenic cleft) have profound effects on T cell recognition either by altering the sites recognized on the MHC class I protein by the TCR complex or by altering the ability of the foreign peptide to be bound appropriately by MHC molecule. In contrast, the determinants recognized on allogeneic MHC molecules remain uncertain. Clearly, the same α-helical residues that interact with antigen-specific T cells determine allogeneic MHC class I recognition. However, the role of processed self or foreign peptides in alloantigen recognition remains unclear. One line of evidence that supports the possibility that peptides may indeed be involved in allogeneic MHC recognition derives from the study of the in vivo and in vitro bm mutants in which a number of amino acids outside the α-helical portions of the α_1/α_2 domain can have a profound effect on T cell recognition. For instance, the bm8 K^b mutations, which are located in the β-pleated sheet, alter allorecognition. Based on the tertiary crystallographic structure of the class I molecule, the distance between these amino acid changes (22, 23, 24) and the surface of the α-helical structures appears too great to cause allosteric effects. It seems more likely that at least a portion of the bm8 anti-K^b alloreactive T cells may recognize self peptides that physically interact with the allogeneic MHC molecule.

The possibility that MHC-specific T cells actually recognize self or foreign peptides in the context of the MHC molecule has profound implications for the development of the T cell repertoire. For instance, T cell tolerance may depend on the recognition of self peptides in the context of self MHC molecules by T cells during thymic development. This possibility is supported by recent studies by Kappler and Marrack [117] in which the clonal deletion of *Vβ17a*-expressing T cells in I-E^k-expressing mice not only depends on the recognition of I-E^k but also tissue-specific peptides. Similarly, Hengartner and colleagues [118] have shown that altered expression T cells utilizing the *Vβ6* gene depends on the appearance of the Mls antigen.

Finally, it is now clear that other regions of the class I molecule play an important role in T cell recognition. Conserved determinants, such as the one dependent on amino acid 227, may not determine MHC specificity but may be instrumental in establishing a functional interaction of the T cell and target cell. It has been suggested that the interaction of CD8 with the class I molecule may be critical in increasing the receptor/ligand avidity. These molecules may both bind MHC antigens on target cells thus helping to specifically stabilize or redistribute the T cell receptor complex during T cell activation or perhaps CD8 molecules deliver a signal themselves. It will be interesting to determine if a similar determinant exists on class II molecules in either the α_2 or β_2 domains that forms a site for CD4 binding.

Acknowledgements

The authors wish to thank Drs. Mark Saper and Donald Wiley for their helpful discussions, insights and data analysis presented in this review. The authors also thank Drs. Bronwyn Houlden and Suzanne Widacki for their helpful discussions and review of the manuscript. Finally, the authors are indebted to the many investigators involved in the studies summarized above. Without the many fruitful collaborations over the years, much of the experimentation summarized above would not have been possible.

References

1 Hood, L.; Steinmetz, M.; Malissen, B.: Genes of the major histocompatibility complex of the mouse. Ann. Rev. Immunol. *1:* 529 (1983).
2 Weiss, E.H.; Golden, L.; Fahrner, K.; Mellor, A.L.; Devlin, J.J.; Bullman, H.; Tiddens, H.; Bud, H.; Flavell, R.A.: Organization and evolution of the class I gene family in the major histocompatibility complex of the C57BL/10 mouse. Nature *310:* 650 (1984).
3 Fisher, D.A.; Hunt, S.W.; Hood, L.: Structure of a gene encoding a murine thymus leukemia antigen, and organization of Tla genes in the BALB/c mouse. J. exp. Med. *162:* 528 (1985).
4 Steinmetz, M.; Winoto, A.; Minard, K.; Hood, L.: Clusters of genes encoding mouse transplantation antigens. Cell *28:* 489 (1982).
5 Klein, J.: H-2 mutations: their genetics and effect on immune functions. Adv. Immunol. *26:* 55 (1978).
6 Zinkernagel, R.M.; Doherty, P.C.: MHC-restricted cytotoxic T cells: studies on the biological role of polymorphic major transplantation antigens determining T-cell restriction-specificity, function, and responsiveness. Adv. Immunol. *27:* 51 (1979).
7 Forman, J.; Goodenow, R.S.; Hood, L.; Ciavarra, R.: Use of DNA-mediated gene transfer to analyze the role of H-2L^d in controlling the specificity of antivesicular stomatitis virus cytotoxic T cells. J. exp. Med. *157:* 1261 (1983).
8 Mizuochi, T.; Ono, S.; Malek, T.R.; Singer, A.: Characterization of two distinct primary T cell populations that secrete interleukin 2 upon recognition of class I or class II major histocompatibility antigens. J. exp. Med. *163:* 603 (1986).
9 Levy, R.B.; Richardson, J.C.; Margulies, D.H.; Evans, G.A.; Seidman, J.G.; Ozato, K.: The products of transferred H-2 genes express determinants that restrict hapten-specific cytotoxic T cells. J. Immun. *130:* 2514 (1983).

10 Flaherty, L.; DiBiase, K.; Lynes, M.A.; Seidman, J.G.; Weinberger, O.; Rinchik, E.M.: Characterization of a Q subregion gene in the murine major histocompatibility complex. Proc. natn. Acad. Sci. USA *82:* 1503 (1985).
11 Weiss, E.H.; Golden, L.; Fahrner, K.; Mellor, A.L.; Devlin, J.J.; Bullman, H.; Tiddens, H.; Bud, H.; Flavell, R.A.: Organization and evolution of the class I gene family in the major histocompatibility complex of the C57BL/10 mouse. Nature *310:* 650 (1984).
12 Chen, Y.-T.; Obata, Y.; Stockert, E.; Takahashi, T.; Old, L.J.: Tla region genes and their products. Immunol. Res. *6:* 30 (1987).
13 Fischer-Lindahl, K.; Bocchieri, M.; Riblet, R.: Maternally transmitted target antigen for unrestricted killing by NZB T lymphocytes. J. exp. Med. *152:* 1583 (1980).
14 Kastner, D.L.; Rich, R.R.; Chu, L: Qa-1-associated antigens. II. Evidence for functional differentiation from H-2K and H-2D antigens. J. Immun. *123:* 1239 (1979).
15 Forman, J.; Trial, J.-A.; Tonkonogy, S.; Flaherty, L.: The Qa2 subregion controls the expression of two antigens recognized by the H-2-unrestricted cytotoxic T cells. J. exp. Med. *155:* 749 (1982).
16 Kimball, E.S.; Coligan, J.E.: Structure of class I major histocompatibility antigens. Contemp. Top. mol. Immunol. *9:* 1–63 (1982).
17 Yokoyama, K.; Geier, S.S.; Uehara, H.; Nathenson, S.F.: Secondary structure of the murine histompatibility alloantigen H-2K^{b}: relationship between heavy chain, beta 2-microglobulin, and antigen reactivity. Biochemistry *24:* 3002 (1985).
18 Ozato, K.; Evans, G.A.; Shykind, B.; Margulies, D.H.; Seidman, J.G.: Hybrid H-2 histocompatibility gene products assign domains recognized by alloreactive T cells. Proc. natn. Acad. Sci. USA *80:* 2040 (1983).
19 Levy, R.B.; Ozato, K.; Richardson, J.C.; Bluestone, J.A.: Molecular localization of allogeneic and self determinants recognized by bulk and clonal populations of cytotoxic T cells. J. Immun. *134:* 677 (1985).
20 Potter, T.A.; Palladino, M.A.; Wilson, D.B.; Rajan, T.W.: Epitopes on H-2D^{d} somatic cell mutants recognized by cytotoxic T cells. J. exp. Med. *158:* 1061 (1983).
21 Bjorkman, P.J.; Saper, M.A.; Samraoui, B.; Bennett, W.S.; Strominger, J.L.; Wiley, D.C.: Structure of the human class I histocompatibility antigen, HLA-A2. Nature *329:* 506 (1987).
22 Shimonkevitz, R.; Kappler, J.; Marrack, P.; Grey, H.: Antigen-recognition by H-2 restricted T cells. I. Cell free antigen processing. J. exp. Med. *158:* 303 (1983).
23 Livingstone, A.M.; Fathman, C.G.: The structure of T-cell epitopes. A. Rev. Immunol. *5:* 477 (1987).
24 Maryanski, J.L.; Pala, P.; Corradin, G.; Jordan, B.R.; Cerottini, J.-C.: H-2-restricted cytolytic T cells specific for HLA can recognize a synthetic HLA peptide. Nature *324:* 578 (1986).
25 Watts, T.H.; Gaub, H.E.; McConnell, H.M.: T cell-mediated association of peptide antigen and major histocompatibility complex protein detected by energy transfer in an evanescent wavefield. Nature *320:* 179 (1986).
26 Buus, S.; Colon, S.; Smith, C.; Freed, J.H.; Miles, C.; Grey, H.M.: Interaction between a 'processed' ovalbumin peptide and Ia molecules. Proc. natn. Acad. Sci. USA *83:* 3968 (1986).
27 Babbitt, B.P.; Allen, P.M.; Matsueda, G.; Haber, E.; Unanue, E.R.: Binding of immunogenic peptides to Ia histocompatibility molecules. Nature *317:* 359–361 (1985).
28 Guillet, J.-G.; Lai, M.-Z.; Briner, T.J.; Buus, S.; Sette, A.; Grey, H.M.; Smith, J.; Gefter, M.L.: Immmunological self, nonself discrimination. Science *235:* 865 (1987).
29 Townsend, A.R.M.; Rothbard, J.; Gotch, F.M.; Bahadur, G.; Wraith, D.; McMichael, A.J.: The epitopes of influenza nucleoprotein recognized by cytotoxic T lymphocytes can be defined with short synthetic peptides. Cell *44:* 959 (1986).

30 Ajitkumar, P.; Geier, S.S.; Kesari, K.V.; Boriello, F.; Nakagawa, M.; Bluestone, J.A.; Saper, M.A.; Wiley, D.C.; Nathenson, S.G.: Evidence that multiple residues on both the α-helices of the class I MHC molecule are simultaneously recognized by the T cell receptor. Cell *54:* 46 (1988).

31 Brown, J.H.; Jardetzky, T.; Saper, M.A.; Samraoui, B.; Bjorkman, P.J.; Wiley, D.C.: A hypothetical model of the foreign antigen binding site of class II histocompatibility molecules. Nature *332:* 845 (1988).

32 Mellor, A.L.; Golden, L.; Weiss, E.; Bullman, H.; Hurst, J.; Simpson, E.; James, R.F.L.; Townsend, A.R.M.; Taylor, P.M.; Schmidt, W.; Ferluga, J.; Leben, L.; Santamaria, M.; Atfield, G.; Festenstein, H.; Flavell, R.A.: Expression of murine H-2Kb histocompatibility antigen in cells transformed with cloned H-2 genes. Nature *298:* 529 (1982).

33 Barbosa, J.A.; Meltzer, S.J.; Minowada, G.; Strominger, J.L.; Burakoff, S.J.; Biro, P.A.: Recognition of HLA-A2 and -B7 antigens by cloned cytotoxic T lymphocytes after gene transfer into human and monkey, but not mouse, cells. Proc. natn. Acad. Sci. USA *81:* 7549 (1984).

34 Evans, G.A.; Margulies, D.H.; Shykind, B.; Seidman, J.G.; Ozato, K.: Exon shuffling: mapping polymorphic determinants on hybrid mouse transplantation antigens. Nature *300:* 755 (1982).

35 Goodenow, R.S.; McMillan, M.; Orn, A.; Nicolson, M.; Davidson, N.; Frelinger, J.A.; Hood, L.: Identification of a BALB/c H-2Ld gene by DNA-mediated gene transfer. Science *215:* 677 (1982).

36 Allen, H.; Wraith, D.; Pala, P.; Askonas, B.; Flavell, R.A.: Domain interactions of H-2 class I antigens alter cytotoxic T-cell recognition sites. Nature *309:* 279 (1984).

37 Stroynowski, I.; Clark, S.; Henderson, L.A.; Hood, L.; McMillan, M.; Forman, J.: Interaction of alpha 1 with alpha 2 region in class I MHC proteins contributes determinants recognized by antibodies and cytotoxic T cells. J. Immun. *135:* 2160 (1985).

38 Stroynowski, I.; Forman, J.; Goodenow, R.S.; Schiffer, S.G.; McMillan, M.; Sharrow, S.O.; Sachs, D.H.; Hood, L.: Expression and T cell recognition of hybrid antigens with amino-terminal domains encoded by Qa-2 region of major histocompatibility complex and carboxyl termini of transplantation antigens. J. exp. Med. *161:* 935 (1985).

39 Stroynowski, I.; Orn, A.; Goodenow, R.S.; McMillian, M.; Forman, J.; Brayton, P.R.; Frelinger, J.; Hood, L.: Cytotoxic T lymphocytes recognize determinants on the BALB/c-H-2L^d molecule controlled by alpha-1 and alpha-2 but not alpha-3 external domains. Immunogenetics *20:* 141 (1984).

40 Arnold, B.; Horstmann, U.; Kuon, W.; Burgert, H.G.; Hammerling, G.J.; Kvist, S.: Alloreactive cytolytic T-cell clones preferentially recognize conformational determinants on histocompatibility antigens: analysis with genetically engineered hybrid antigens. Proc. natn. Acad. Sci. USA *82:* 7030 (1985).

41 Arnold, B.; Burgert, H.G.; Hamann, U.; Hammerling, G.; Kees, U.; Kvist, S.: Cytolytic T cells recognize the two amino-terminal domains of H-2K antigens in tandem in influenza A infected cells. Cell *38:* 79 (1984).

42 Murre, C.; Choi, E.; Weis, J.; Seidman, J.G.; Ozato, K.; Liu, L.; Burakoff, S.J.; Reiss, C.S.: Dissection of serological and cytolytic T lymphocyte epitopes on murine major histocompatibility antigens by a recombinant H-2 gene separating the first two external domains. J. exp. Med. *160:* 167 (1984).

43 Reiss, C.S.; Greenstein, J.L.; Crimmins, M.A.; Liu, L.L.; Rao, A.; Maziarz, R.T.; Murre, C.; Burakoff, S.J.: Recognition of the alpha-1 and alpha-2 domains of H-2 molecules by allospecific cloned T cells. J. Immun. *136:* 2191 (1986).

44 Ozato, K.; Evans, G.A.; Margulies, D.H.; Seidman, J.G.; Levy, R.B.: The use of hybrid H-2 genes for localizing the positions of polymorphic determinants recognized by antibodies and by cytotoxic T cells. Transplant. Proc. *15:* 2074 (1983).

45 Reiss, C.S.; Evans, G.A.; Margulies, D.H.; Seidman, J.G.; Burakoff, S.J.: Allospecific and virus-specific cytolytic T lymphocytes are restricted to the N or C1 domain of H-2 antigens expressed on L cells after DNA-mediated gene transfer. Proc. natn. Acad. Sci. USA *80:* 2709 (1983).
46 Evans, G.A.; Margulies, D.H.; Shykind, B.; Seidman, J.G.; Ozato, L.: Exon shuffling: mapping polymorphic determinants on hybrid mouse transplantation antigens. Nature *300:* 755 (1982).
47 Bluestone, J.A.; Foo, M.; Allen, H.; Flavell, R.A.: Allospecific cytolytic T lymphocytes recognize conformational determinants on hybrid mouse transplantation antigens. J. exp. Med. *162:* 268 (1985).
48 McCluskey, J.; Boyd L.; Foo, M.; Forman, J.; Margulies, D.H.; Bluestone, J.A.: Analysis of hybrid H-2D and L antigens with reciprocally mismatched aminoterminal domains: functional T cell recognition requires preservation of fine structural determinants. J. Immun. *137:* 3881–3890 (1986).
49 Maziarz, R.; Allen, H.; Strominger, J.L.; Flavell, R.; Biro, P.A.; Burakoff, S.J.: Recognition of interspecies hybrid class I histocompatibility antigens by antigen-specific cytolytic T lymphocytes. Proc. natn. Acad. Sci. USA *82:* 6276 (1985).
50 Ozato, K.; Evans, G.A.; Shykind, B.; Margulies, D.H.; Seidman, J.G.: Hybrid H-2 histocompatibility gene products assign domains recognized by alloreactive T cells. Proc. natn. Acad. Sci. USA *80:* 2040 (1983).
51 Ozato, K.; Evans, G.A.; Margulies, D.H.; Seidman, J.G.; Levy, R.B.: The use of hybrid H-2 genes for localizing the positions of polymorphic determinants recognized by antibodies and by cytotoxic T cells. Transplant. Proc. *15:* 2074 (1983).
52 Levy, R.B.; Richardson, J.C.; Margulies, D.H.; Evans, G.A.; Seidman, J.G.; Ozato, K.: The products of transferred H-2 genes express determinants that restrict hapten-specific cytotoxic T cells. J. Immun. *130:* 2514 (1983).
53 Levy, R.B.; Ozato, K.; Richman, J.C.; Bluestone, J.A.: Molecular localization of allogenic and self determinants recognized by bulk and clonal populations of cytotoxic T-cells. J. Immun. *134:* 1342–1348 (1985).
54 Sun, Y.H.; Goodenow, R.S.; Hood, L.: Molecular basis of the dm1 mutation in the major histocompatibility complex of the mouse: a D/L hybrid gene. J. exp. Med. *162:* 1588 (1985).
55 Burnside, S.S.; Hunt, P.; Ozato, K.; Sears, D.W.: A molecular hybrid of the H-2Dd and H-2Ld genes expressed in the dm1 mutant. Proc. natn. Acad. Sci. USA *81:* 5204 (1984).
56 Holmes, N.; Parham, P.: Exon shuffling in vivo can generate novel HLA class I molecules. EMBO J. *4:* 2849 (1985).
57 Clayberger, C.; Holmes, N.; Wang, P.L.; Koller, T.D.; Parham, P.; Krensky, A.M.: Determinants recognized by human cytotoxic T cells on a natural hybrid class I HLA molecule. J. exp. Med. *162:* 1709 (1985).
58 Scholler, J.; Shimonkevitz, R.; MacDonald, H.R.; Kvist, S.: Different structural constraints for recognition of mouse H-2Kd and -Kk antigens by alloimmune cytolytic T lymphocytes. J. exp. Med. *164:* 1823 (1986).
59 Abastado, J.-P.; Jaulin, C.; Schutze, M.-P.; Langlade-Demoyen, P.; Plata, F.; Ozato, K.; Kourilsky, P.: Fine mapping of epitopes by intradomain K^d/D^d recombinants. J. exp. Med. *166:* 327 (1987).
60 Bailey, D.W.; Kohn, H.I.: Inherited histocompatibility changes in progeny of irradiated and unirradiated inbred mice. Genet. Res. *6:* 330 (1975).
61 Egorov, I.K.: A mutation of histocompatibility-2 locus in mouse Genetika *3:* 18 (1977).
62 Melvold, R.W.; Kohn, H.I.: Eight new histocompatibility mutations associated with the H-2 complex. Immunogenetics *3:* 285 (1976).

63 Melvold, R.W.; Kohn, H.I.; Dunn, G.R.: History and genealogy of the H-$2K^b$ mutants from the C57BL-6Kh colony. Immunogenetics *15:* 177 (1982).
64 Egorov, D.S.; Egorov, I.K.: H-2^{bm23}, and new K^b mutant similar to but not identical with H-2^{bm3}. Immunogenetics *20:* 83 (1984).
65 Nathenson, S.G.; Geliebter, J.; Pfaffenbach, G.M.; Zeff, R.A.: Murine major histocompatibility complex class I mutants: molecular analysis and structure-function implications. A. Rev. Immunol. *4:* 471–502 (1986).
66 McKenzie, I.F.C.; Pang, T.; Blanden, R.V.: The use of H-2 mutants as models for the study of T cell activation. Immunol. Rev. *35:* 181 (1977).
67 Melief, C.J.; Waal, L.P. de; Meulen, M.Y. van der; Melvold, R.W.; Kohn, H.I.: Fine specificity of alloimmune cytotoxic T lymphocytes directed against H-2K. A study with K^b mutants. J. exp. Med. *151:* 993 (1980).
68 Weyland, C.; Hammerling, G.J.; Goronzy, J.: Recognition of H-2 domains by cytotoxic T lymphocytes. Nature *292:* 627 (1981).
69 Sherman, L.A.: Mutationally derived H-2 antigenic differences as defined by cytolytic T-lymphocyte clones. J. Immun. *127:* 1259 (1981).
70 Sherman, L.A.: Recognition of conformational determinants on H-2 by cytolytic T lymphocytes. Nature *297:* 511 (1982).
71 Pan, S.; Wettstein, P.J.; Knowles, B.B.: H-$2K^b$ mutations limit the CTL response to SV40 TASA. J. Immun. *128:* 243 (1982).
72 Melief, C.J.M.; Stukart, M.J.; Waal, L. P. de; Kast, W.M.; Melvold, R.W.: Specificity and regulation of cytotoxic T-lymphocyte responses analyzed with H-2 mutants. Transplant. Proc. *15:* 2086 (1983).
73 Davignon, J.L.; Guimezanes, A.; Schmitt-Verhulst, A.M.: Clonal analysis of H-$2K^b$ + TNP recognition by T cells with the use of H-$2K^{bm}$ mutants and H-$2K^b$-specific monoclonal antibodies. J. Immun. *131:* 1073 (1983).
74 Hurwitz, J.L.; Wettstein, P.J.; Bennink, J.R.; Doherty, P.C.: Cross-reactivity patterns of influenza-specific cytotoxic T lymphocytes from H-$2K^b$ mutant mice. J. Immun. *131:* 471 (1983).
75 Hurwitz, J.L.; Pan, S.; Wettstein, P.J.; Doherty, P.C.: Cross-reactivity patterns of vaccinia-specific cytotoxic T lymphocytes from H-$2K^b$ mutants. Immunogenetics *17:* 79 (1983).
76 Byrne, J.A.; Ahmed, R.; Oldstone, M.B.: Biology of cloned cytotoxic T lymphocytes specific for lymphocytic choriomeningitis virus. I. Generation and recognition of virus strains and H-2^b mutants. J. Immun. *133:* 433 (1984).
77 Stukart, M.J.; Boes, J.; Melief, C.J.: Recognition of H-$2K^b$ mutant target cells by Moloney virus-specific cytotoxic T lymphocytes from bm13 (H-$2D^b$-mutant) mice. II. Relationship of K^{bm3} and K^{bm11} in restriction specificities and allodeterminants. J. Immun. *113:* 28 (1984).
78 Bluestone, J.A.; Palman, C.; Foo, M.; Geier, S.S.; Nathenson, S.G.: Analysis of major histocompatibility complex class 1 antigens using in vitro-derived somatic cell mutants; in Sercarz, Cantor, Chess, Regulation of the immune system. UCLA Symp. on Molecular and Cellular Biology (new ser.) vol. 18, pp. 89–97 (Liss, New York 1984).
79 Martinko, J.M.; Solheim, J.C.; Geliebter, J.: The H-$2K^{km1}$ mutation: a single nucleotide substitution is responsible for multiple functional differences in a class I MHC molecule. Mol. Immunol. *25:* 267 (1988).
80 Vohr, H.W.; Holtkamp, B.; Rajewsky, K.: Somatic H-$2K^k$ variants reveal nonidentity of serological and cytotoxic T cells. Eur. J. Immunol. *13:* 846 (1984).
81 Mellor, A.L.; Weiss, E.H.; Ramachandran, K.; Flavell, R.A.: A potential donor gene for the bm1 gene conversion event in the C57BL mouse. Nature *306:* 792 (1983).

82 Weiss, E.H.; Mellor, A.; Golden, L.; Fahrner, K.; Simpson, E.; Hurst, J.; Flavell, R.A.: The structure of a mutant H-2 gene suggests that the generation of polymorphism in H-2 genes may occur by gene conversion-like events. Nature *301:* 671 (1983).

83 Schulze, D.H.; Pease, L.R.; Yokoyama, K.; Geier, S.S.; Pfaffenbach, G.M.; Geliebter, J.; Zeff, R.A.; Rosenblatt, B.P.; Nathenson, S.G.: Diversity and polymorphism in the MHC appear to be generated by a copy mechanism. Transplant. Proc. *15:* 2009 (1983).

84 Schulze, D.H.; Pease, L.R.; Geier, S.S.; Reyes, A.A.; Sarmiento, L.A.; Wallace, R.B.; Nathenson, S.G.: Comparison of the cloned H-$2K^{bm1}$ variant gene with the H-$2K^{b}$ gene shows a cluster of seven nucleotide differences. Proc. natn. Acad. Sci. USA *80:* 2007 (1983).

85 Geier, S.S.; Zeff, R.A.; McGovern, D.M.; Rajan, T.V.; Nathenson, S.G.: An approach to the study of structure-function relationships of MHC class I molecules: isolation and serologic characterization of H-$2K^{b}$ somatic cell variants. J. Immun. *137:* 1239 (1986).

86 Lewis, J.; Foo, M.; Geier, S.S.; Ajitkumar, P.; Nathenson, S.G.; Bluestone, J.A.: CTL recognition of novel allodeterminants expressed on in vitro-selected H-$2K^{b}$ mutants. J. Immun. *141:* 728 (1988).

87 Morgan, G.M.; McKenzie, I.J.; Melvold, R.W.: Studies of H-$2K^{b}$ mutant mice. II. Definition of new H-2 specificities (H-2.68, 69, 71, 72) using the H-$2K^{b}$ mutant, B6.C-H-2^{bm10}. Immunogenetics *11:* 43 (1980).

88 Sherman, L.A.; Randolph, C.P.: Monoclonal anti-H-$2K^{b}$ antibodies detect serological differences between H-$2K^{b}$ mutants. Immunogenetics *12:* 183 (1981).

89 Hammerling, G.J.; Rush, E.; Tada, N.; Kimura, S.; Hammerling, U.: Localization of allodeterminants on H-$2K^{b}$ antigens determined with monoclonal antibodies and H-2 mutant mice. Proc. natn. Acad. Sci. USA *79:* 4737 (1982).

90 Bluestone, J.A.; McKenzie, I.F.; Melvold, R.W.; Ozato, K.; Sandrin, M.S.; Sharrow, S.O.; Sachs, D.H.: Serological analysis of H-2 mutations using monoclonal antibodies. J. Immunogenet. *11:* 197 (1984).

91 Bjorkman, P.J.; Saper, M.A.; Samraoui, B.; Bennett, W.S.; Strominger, J.L.; Wiley, D.C.: The foreign antigen binding site and T cell recognition regions of class I histocompatibility antigens. Nature *329:* 512 (1987).

92 Geier, S.S.; Zeff, R.A.; Rajan, T.V.; Nathenson, S.G.: Analysis of K^{b} somatic cell variants: an approach to the study of MHC structure-function relationships. J. Immun. *137:* 1239 (1986).

93 Holtkamp, B.; Cramer, M.; Lemke, H.; Rajewsky, K.: Isolation of a cloned cell line expressing variant H-$2K^{k}$ using fluorescence-activated cell sorting. Nature *289:* 66 (1981).

94 Rajan, T.V.; Halay, E.D.: Anti-H-2 hybridoma antibodies as immunoselective agents. I. Isolation of forward and reverse mutations for reactivity with a monoclonal antibody. Immunogenetics *14:* 253 (1981).

95 Bluestone, J.A.; Langlet C.; Geier, S.S.; Nathenson, S.G.; Foo, M.; Schmitt-Verhulst, A.-M.: Somatic cell variants express altered H-$2K^{b}$ allodeterminants recognized by cytolytic T cell clones. J. Immun. *137:* 1244 (1986).

96 Nakagawa, M.; Zeff, R.A.; Geier, S.S.; Bluestone, J.A.; Nathenson, S.G.: Somatic cell variants of H-2Kb: a point mutation in the first extracellular domain results in altered recognition. Immunogenetics *24:* 381 (1986).

97 Horstmann, U.; Arnold, B.; Hammerling, G.J.: Unrestricted recognition of class I neodeterminants generated by exon shuffling. Eur. J. Immunol. *16:* 863 (1986).

98 Kanda, T.; LaPan, K.; Takahashi, H.; Appella, E.; Frelinger, J.A.: The alpha1 and alpha2 domains of H-2 class I molecules interact to form unique epitopes. Immunogenetics *25:* 110 (1987).

99 Koeller, D.; Lieberman, R.; Miyazaki, J.; Appella, E.; Ozato, K.; Mann, D.W.; Forman, J.: Introduction of H-2Dd determinants into the H-2Ld antigen by site-directed mutagenesis. J. exp. Med. *166:* 744 (1987).
100 Maziarz, R.; Allen, H.; Strominger, J.; Flavell, D.; Bird, P.A.; Burakoff, S.: Recognition of interspecies hybrid class I histocompatibility antigens by antigen-specific cytolytic T lymphocytes. Proc. natn. Acad. Sci. USA. *82:* 6276 (1985).
101 Maziarz, R.T.; Burakoff, S.J.; Bluestone, J.A.: Interdependence of the polymorphic domains of the class I MHC molecule on the constant domains as determined by CTL recognition. J. Immun. *140:* 4372 (1988).
102 McCluskey, J.; Bluestone, J.A.; Coligan, J.E.; Maloy, W.L.; Margulies, D.H.: Serologic and T cell recognition of truncated transplantation antigens encoded by in vitro deleted class I major histocompatibility genes. J. Immun. *136:* 1472–1481 (1986).
103 Ciavarra, R.; Forman, J.: H-2L-restricted recognition of viral antigens in the H-2d haplotype, anti-vesicular stomatitis virus cytotoxic T cells are restricted solely by H-2L. J. exp. Med. *156:* 778 (1982).
104 Potter, T.A.; Hansen, T.H.; Habbersett, R.; Ozato, K.; Ahmed, A.: Flow microfluorometric analysis of H2L expression. J. Immun. *127:* 580 (1981).
105 Connolly, J.M.; Potter, T.A.; Wormstall, E.-M.; Hansen, T.H.: The Lyt-2 molecule recognizes residues in the class I alpha 3 domain in allogeneic cytolytic T cell responses. J. exp. Med. *168:* 325 (1988).
106 Bluestone, J.A.; Potter, T.A.; Chatterjee-Hasrouni, S.; Rajan, T.V.: CTL recognize different determinants from those defined serologically on Ld somatic cell mutants. J. Immun. *133:* 1168–1173 (1984).
107 Potter, T.A.; Palladino, M.A.; Wilson, D.B.; Rajan, T.V.: Epitopes on H-2D^d somatic cell mutants recognized by cytotoxic T cells. J. exp. Med. *158:* 1061 (1983).
108 Potter, T.A.; Bluestone, J.A.; Rajan, T.V.: A single amino acid substitution in the α_3 domain of an H-2 class I molecule abrogates reactivity with CTL. J. exp. Med. *166:* 956 (1987).
109 Potter, T.A.; Rajan, T.V.; Dick, R.F.; Bluestone, J.A.: Substitution at residue 227 of H-2 class I molecules abrogates recognition by CD8-dependent, but not CD8 independent, CTL. Nature *337:* 735 (1989).
110 Swain, S.L.: T cell subsets and the recognition of class I. Immunol. Rev. *74:* 129 (1983).
111 Swain, S.L.: Significance of Lyt phenotypes: Lyt-2 antibodies block activates of T cells that recognize class I major histocompatibility antigens regardless of their function. Proc. natn. Acad. Sci. USA *78:* 7101 (1981).
112 Dembic, Z.; Haas, W.; Zamoyska, R.; Parnes, J.; Steinmetz, M.; Boehmer, H. von: Transfection of the CD8 gene enhances T cell recognition. Nature *326:* 510 (1987).
113 Gabert, J.; Langlet, C.; Zamoyska, R.; Parnes, J.R.; Schmitt-Verhulst, A.-M.; Malissen, B.: Reconstitution of MHC class I specificity by transfer of the T cell receptor and Lyt-2 genes. Cell *50:* 545 (1987).
114 MacDonald, H.R.; Glasebrook, A.L.; Bron, C.; Kelsoe, A.; Cerottini, J.-C.: Clonal heterogeneity in the functional requirement for Lyt 2, 3 molecules on cytotoxic T lymphocytes (CTL): possible implications for the affinity of CTL antigen receptors. Immunol. Rev. *68:* 89 (1982).
115 Amit, A.G.; Mariuzza, R.A.; Phillips, S.E.V.; Poljak, R.J.: Three-dimensional structure of an antigen-antibody complex at 2.8 A resolution. Science *233:* 747 (1986).
116 Getzoff, E.D.; Tainer, J.A.; Lerner, R.A.; Geysen, H.M.: The chemistry and mechanism of antibody binding to protein antigens. Adv. Immunol. *43:* 1 (1988).

117 Kappler, J.W.; Wade, T.; White, J.; Kushnir, E.; Blackman, M.; Bill, J.; Roehm, N.; Marrack, P.: A T cell receptor V beta segment that imparts reactivity to a class II major histocompatibility complex product. Cell *49:* 263–271 (1987).
118 MacDonald, H.R.; Schneider, R.; Lees, R.K.; Howe, R.C.; Acha-Orbea, H.; Festenstein, H.; Zinkernagel, R.M.; Hengartner, H.: T-cell receptor V beta use predicts reactivity and tolerance to Mls^{a}-encoded antigens. Nature *332:* 40 (1988).

Jeffrey A. Bluestone, PhD, Ben May Institute, University of Chicago, Chicago, IL 60637 (USA)

Sercarz E (ed): Antigenic Determinants and Immune Regulation. Chem Immunol.
Basel, Karger, 1989, vol 46, pp 49–84

Structural Requirements for Class II Molecule Recognition by Antibodies and T Cell Antigen Receptors

David J. McKean[1]

Department of Immunology, Mayo Clinic, Rochester, Minn., USA

Introduction

T lymphocytes that express the CD4 surface marker play a key role in the generation of an antigen specific immune response. Once activated, these lymphocytes produce a number of cytokines that are directly or indirectly responsible for the activation, clonal expansion and differentiation of B lymphocytes, cytotoxic T lymphocytes and a variety of other cells that participate in an inflammatory response. $CD4^{+}$ T lymphocytes become activated once their cell surface antigen receptors (T_R) bind to and are cross-linked by an appropriate ligand. The ligand bound by these T_R does not consist of native antigen but is a complex comprised of antigen fragments bound to self class II (Ia) molecules. This article will review recent studies that have helped elucidate how Ia molecules function to generate an appropriate ligand capable of binding to a T_R. Most of this article will focus on studies using molecular techniques to identify the functional regions on the murine class II molecule. Although studies concerning the derivation and chemical nature of the antigen fragment will be summarized, detailed reviews of the experiments that are the basis for the currently accepted view of this area have been published recently [1, 2]. Studies elucidating the nature of antibody binding sites on the murine class II molecule also will be analyzed in order to obtain additional information about how another receptor, which is evolutionarily related to the T_R, binds to the Ia molecule. Finally, since structural diversity is generated by the interaction of polymorphic residues on different pairs of class II α and

[1] I am very grateful to Drs. Barbara Beck and Larry Pease for their critical reading of this manuscript. I would also like to thank Therese Lee for her skilled assistance in the preparation of the manuscript.

β polypeptides, recent studies exploring the molecular basis for allele specific associations of the two polypeptide chains will be discussed.

Antigen Presentation and the Characterization of Immunogenic Peptides

It was recognized in the 1960s that, unlike B lymphocytes, T lymphocytes do not discriminate between native and denatured antigen [3–5]. In the early 1970s, Mosier [6] demonstrated that T lymphocytes were incapable of recognizing soluble antigen and only recognized antigens in the presence of antigen-presenting cells (APC). Subsequently, these APC were shown to present antigen that had been internalized and 'processed' by a temperature- and time-dependent process [7, 8]. Our understanding of the molecular events involved in this process was enhanced when Rosenthal and Shevach [9] demonstrated that molecules encoded in the major histocompatibility complex (MHC) were involved in restricting the interaction between T lymphocytes and APC. Specifically, primed antigen reactive T cells would respond to the appropriate antigen only when presented by syngeneic class II bearing APC and not when presented by allogeneic APC. Earlier studies from the laboratories of Benacerraf and McDevitt [10–12] had demonstrated that inbred strains of animals produced either high or low titers of antibody when challenged with certain synthetic antigens. Together, these analyses led to the development of the concept that the class II molecules on the surface of the APC were directly involved in presenting antigen to the T lymphocyte. Rosenthal [13] coined the term 'determined selection' to describe the hypothesis that the class II molecule could determine which portion of the antigen was preferentially recognized by the T lymphocyte.

Although it was apparent that antigen processing involved the degradation of antigen, the identification of the biologically relevant antigenic moiety proved to be a very difficult task. Radiolabeled antigen fragments could be isolated from APC extracts, but it was impossible to determine which fragment was the biologically relevant material. A significant advance was made when Ziegler and Unanue [14] treated APC with paraformaldehyde to crosslink their surface proteins and prevent exo- and endocytosis. Aldehyde fixed cells could present antigen that had been cultured with the APC prior to fixation but were unable to present antigen cultured with the APC after fixation. These results demonstrated that after a limited obligatory processing period the appropriate ligand for the T cell receptor was present on the surface of the APC. Shimonkevitz et al. [15] then demonstrated that fixed APC were capable of presenting tryptic fragments of antigen to T cells. This 'cell free antigen processing' showed that a degraded form of the antigen could associate with class II molecules on the surface of a fixed APC and the resulting complex could be recognized effectively by the T cell receptor. This observation confirmed previous results demonstrating that antigen processing involved the internalization and degradation of the antigen molecules. More importantly, it established an experimental system in which an extrinsically processed antigen fragment could associate effectively with class II molecules on the surface of a fixed APC and the resulting complex could be recognized by a T cell receptor. This model system has been used by a number of investigators to identify the minimal fragment of an antigen that will function as an antigenic determinant for T cell recognition. For most antigens, this determinant is comprised of a linear sequence of ten to twelve amino acids. A limited number of antigens have been identified that apparently do not need to be degraded/denatured before they associate with class II molecules and are recognized by the T cell receptor [16, 17]. These exceptions may be due to particular secondary structural features of certain antigens.

Another significant advance in the characterization of the antigen-class II interaction resulted from the observations of Babbitt et al. [18] who demonstrated that detergent solubilized class II molecules would bind appropriate antigenic peptides in solution. Using similar techniques, a number of laboratories have demonstrated that, in general, these immunogenic peptides bind to soluble class II molecules from responder but not nonresponder strains [reviewed in ref. 1]. Peptide binding to class II molecules is a saturable process with an affinity in the micromolar range [19]. However, in solution, association rate constants ($1.2\ M^{-1}\ s^{-1}$) and dissociation rate constants (10^{-5} to $10^{-6}\ s^{-1}$) are relatively slow considering the biological requirements on the APC. If the rate constants measured in solution are representative of the rate constants that occur in the APC, then the class II molecule and processed antigen fragment need to be spatially adjacent and in relatively high concentrations for a considerable length of time in order to obtain association. This association could potentially occur in endocytic vesicles containing class II molecules derived from the plasma membrane [20] and antigen that has been internalized by either receptor-mediated endocytosis or pinocytosis. Once bound, the peptide-class II complex would have $T\frac{1}{2}$ of 5–10 h at 37 °C [1]. Potential problems related to the saturation of the existing class II molecules with processed antigen could be obviated if the dissociation rate is enhanced at the low pH of the endocytic vesicle as the class II-processed antigen complex cycles from the plasma membrane to the endocytic vesicles and back to the plasma membrane.

The immunogenic peptide-class II molecule solution-binding assay also permitted the development of experiments measuring competitive binding of antigen fragments to a single allelic form of the class II molecule [1, 18, 21]. Antigenic competition has been shown to take place only among peptides that are presented to T cells by the same restriction element (class II allele). These results are consistent with the determinant selection hypothesis. However, there are examples in which antigenic fragments bind to class II molecules that are not restricting elements for T cell activation [2, 22]. These results could be explained in the context of the biological system if nonresponsiveness can be generated when the T cells, which are capable of reacting with this particular peptide-class II complex, are deleted during T cell maturation. Such T cells would be deleted during ontogeny if the antigenic determinant resembles a self determinant. This process of generating specific antigen nonresponsiveness has been referred to as the 'hole in the repertoire' [23] and is an alternative to the determinant selection mechanism for regulating T cell specificity.

The observation that different antigenic fragments bind in a competitive manner to the same class II molecule indicates that the class II molecule has a single functional binding site [18, 24]. These results are consistent with the recently published analysis of the class I crystal structure that showed one potential binding site in the most membrane-distal domain of the molecule [25, 26]. If the antigenic fragment binds to a single site, then it should be possible to use alternative forms of the antigen fragment to identify which amino acids are important for binding to the class II molecule and which are important for T cell receptor recognition [23, 27, 28]. In addition, it should be possible to identify the structural constraints imposed by the T cell receptor binding site on the antigen processing mechanism.

The biochemical basis of the association between the antigenic fragment and class II molecules or T_R is an area of active investigation in a number of laboratories. A number of hypotheses have been proposed on the basis of results with different model systems. It has been proposed that the antigenic peptide assumes an alpha-helical or amphipathic α-helical structure in order to bind in the class II antigen-binding site [29]. In computer modeling analyses with some antigens, residues that have been mapped by competition studies to associate with the class II binding site are located on one side of the α helix and residues that have been mapped to associate with the T_R are located on the other side of the α helix [2]. However, the α helix motif may not be shared by all antigens [1, 30]. Although there may not be a single peptide structural motif required for effective association with the T_R binding site, class II allele-specific structural patterns do seem to be shared between a number of different antigenic determinants [28]. Peptides may be particularly immunogenic because they can form an α helix and they have residues located on one face of the helix capable of interacting with allele specific residues in the class II antigen-binding site. Further refinement of these studies that combine computer modeling and direct binding analyses of synthetic peptides to purified class II molecules should lead to the development of effective strategies to produce antagonists that can modulate particular antigen specific immune responses.

Class II Molecular Characterization

Two isotypic forms of murine class II molecules, designated A and E, are encoded in the I region of the MHC. Both isotypic forms are polymorphic integral membrane glycoproteins, consisting of a 33-kilodalton α polypeptide noncovalently associated with a 29-kilodalton β polypeptide. Both the α and β polypeptides contain two extracellular domains of approximately 96 amino acids, designated α_1 and α_2, β_1 and β_2, respectively [31]. The genes encoding the murine class II α and β polypeptides exhibit similar intron-exon organization. The α chain genes are divided into five exons that encode the leader sequence, the α_1 domain, the α_2 domain, the transmembrane/cytoplasmic domain and the 3′ untranslated region [32]. The β chain gene is divided into six exons that encode the leader segment and first few residues of the β_1 domain, the β_1 domain, the β_2 domain, the transmembrane domain, the cytoplasmic domain and last few residues of the cytoplasmic domain plus the 3′ untranslated region [33].

Both polypeptides contain N-linked oligosaccharides which are variably sialylated, resulting in charge heterogeneity of both polypeptides. The α and β polypeptides are synthesized in the endoplasmic reticulum as 28- and 26-kilodalton polypeptides that associate in a trimolecular complex with a 21-kilodalton nonpolymorphic invariant (I_i) polypeptide, which is not encoded in the MHC [34]. Although the function of the I_i polypeptide is unknown, its intracellular association with class II polypeptides suggests that it may function in the intracellular transport of class II molecules [35, 36]. However, several studies have demonstrated that class II molecules can be expressed, albeit inefficiently, in cells that do not express the I_i polypeptide [37, 38]. Although it is not known how it associates with the class II molecule, recent evidence from a class II expression variant indicates that the I_i polypeptide can associate with the β chain in the absence of the α chain [39]. As the heterotrimer moves through the Golgi, complex oligosaccharides and sialic acid are added to each of the three polypeptides. The I_i polypeptide dissociates from the α-β complex before the fully glycosylated class II heterodimer moves from the trans face of the Golgi to the plasma membrane [40]. The class II molecules on the plasma membrane are then cycled between the endocytic vesicles and the plasma membrane. Presumably, during the time when the class II molecules cycle through the endocytic vesicles, these molecules bind antigenic fragments that have been produced by proteolytic degradation in the intracytoplasmic vesicles. Class II molecules are not 'processed' in the endocytic vesicles at least, in part, because the molecules are relatively resistant to proteolysis.

Nearly all of what we know about α and β chain protein sequences has been deduced from sequencing class II genes. The proteins are expressed at such low levels in cells that conventional protein sequence analysis of the molecules was not practical. Sequence analysis of allelic α and β chain genes revealed that most polymorphic residues are located in the NH_2-terminal α_1 and β_1 domains [reviewed in ref. 41]. These polymorphic residues tend to be clustered in three or four regions of the primary structure in both NH_2-terminal domains. The clusters of polymorphic residues were hypothesized to comprise the immunogenic peptide binding sites [41]. Because of their potential structure-function homology to immunoglobulin hypervariable regions, the class II polymorphic residue clusters have been referred to as class II hypervariable regions by some investigators [41]. However, unlike immunoglobulin hypervariable regions, the variability in the class II clusters is not generated by somatic mutation. In addition, the role of the regions in binding foreign antigen has yet to be proven. In this review I will refer to these class II regions as polymorphic regions, in keeping with their genetic origin.

Class II Gene Transfer and Expression

The isolation and sequence analysis of the class II genes opened up a new approach that has greatly facilitated the structure-function analysis of class II molecules. Prior to this discovery, very little direct information relating structure to function was available. Clearly, the major obstacle to this analysis was the difficulties involved in obtaining the relatively large amount of class II protein needed for conventional biochemical analysis. Prior to 1981, both functional and biochemical analyses of class II molecules were carried out on material isolated from heterogeneous populations of splenocytes, lymph node cells or peritoneal macrophages. These cells were obtained from animals and expressed relatively low levels of class II molecules. In 1981, cloned, B lymphoma cell lines were shown to be efficient APC [42]. These cells express high levels of class II molecules and can be grown in large numbers in vitro. Although B lymphoma cells were useful for the initial biochemical analyses of class II molecules, large scale preparation of class II molecules for protein sequence analysis was unnecessary due to technological advances in gene cloning and sequencing procedures. As will be described later, the use of B lymphoma cells in combination with DNA-mediated gene transfer has provided a valuable model system for the molecular characterization of the role of class II molecules in T lymphocyte activation.

In 1983, several different laboratories reported the transfection and stable expression of human and mouse class II genes in class II negative murine L cells or allele mismatched, class II bearing B lymphoma cell lines [43–46]. Genomic clones of α and β genes, together with a gene encoding a selectable marker (thymidine kinase, xanthine-guanine phosphoribosyl transferase), were transfected into target cells using either calcium phosphate precipitation or spheroplast fusion. Transformants were isolated by culturing the cells in a selection medium (hypoxanthine-aminopterin-thymidine or mycophenolic acid-xanthine). Surface expression of the class II molecules required the transfection of both α and β genes. In both human and mouse gene transfection experiments, class II expression was obtained in mouse L cells whether or not the I_i gene was cotransfected with the α and β genes [44, 46]. Although not known at that time, L cells have since been reported to express an endogenous I_i polypeptide and the mouse I_i polypeptide [47] has been shown to associate with either mouse or human intracellular class II molecules [48]. The class II molecules expressed by the transfected cells were determined to be normal by biochemical and serologic criteria. However, L cells expressed low levels of class II molecules as compared with the levels observed on B lymphoma cells [49].

Since the principal biologic function of class II molecules is to be a component of the ligand (restriction element) for the T lymphocyte antigen receptor, it was important to determine if class II transfected cells could process and present antigen to T cells. The class II transfected cell lines were capable of presenting a variety of soluble antigens to the appropriate antigen reactive T hybridomas [49, 50]. This result indicated that the ability to process antigen was not a unique function of B cells and macrophages but rather is probably a normal component of the endocytic process. However, the transfected cells were unable to present antigen to some antigen reactive T cell clones [49, 50]. This result may, in part, be due to the fact that T cell hybridomas have less stringent activation requirements than do T cell clones. Since at least some transfected L cell lines express lower levels of class II molecules on their surface, they may not be able to cross-link sufficient numbers of T cell antigen receptors on the T cell clones to initiate the activation program. In addition, L cells may not express appropriate accessory molecules that may be ligands for T lymphocyte auxiliary receptors, which function to enhance cell-cell interactions or to initiate additional activation signals during the APC-T cell interaction.

Lechler et al. [51] demonstrated that anti-LFA-1 antibodies, which are potent inhibitors of T cell activation in the presence of B lymphoma APC, have no effect on T cell activation mediated by transfected L cell APC. Although the mechanism responsible for this anti-LFA-1-mediated inhibition is unknown, the results support the hypothesis that L cells may be deficient in some of the accessory functions that may be important for the activation of at least some T cells.

As will be discussed in a later section, a number of laboratories now avoid the potential problems associated with the use of L cells as APC by transfecting class II genes into class II negative B lymphoma cells [52, 53]. These transfected B lymphoma cells are, by the criteria outlined above, fully competent APC. In addition, it should be mentioned that the techniques for transfecting class II genes into cells have improved significantly since 1983. Unlike the original procedures used to transfect genes, the introduction of foreign class II genes into cells is now a highly reproducible technique. As long as the cells are cultured in selection medium, the levels of cell surface class II expression are very stable, even after months of in vitro culture. A variety of plasmids encoding additional selectable markers (neomycin, hygromycin) are readily available and electroporation techniques have largely replaced other procedures for the introduction of foreign genes into many different cell types. Cells can be sequentially transfected with a variety of combinations of genes and selectable markers [37].

Class II Mutants – Serologic and T Cell Receptor Epitopes

In-vivo-Derived Mutant

Although the B6.C-H-2^{bm12} (bm12) is the only spontaneous class II mutant identified, its biological characterization demonstrated the potential knowledge that could be gained by studying class II variants. The bm12 mutant was shown to be of the gain and loss type when parent and mutant strains reciprocally rejected skin grafts [54]. The mutation resulted in both the loss of serologic epitopes and in altered T cell antigen recognition (Ir gene phenotype) [55, 56]. The altered class II phenotype was later characterized to be due to three substitutions (positions 67, 70 and 71) in the A_β^b β_1 domain [57]. The substitutions potentially resulted from a gene conversion-like event in which E_β^b sequence was transferred to the A_β^b gene [58, 59].

In-vitro-Derived Mutants – Immunoselected

Two general types of in-vitro-derived class II mutants have been produced in a number of laboratories. One type of mutant was immunoselected from mutagenized class II-bearing B lymphoma cells and the second type was produced by genetic engineering.

The immunoselected class II mutants were produced by treating ethylmethane sulfonate-treated B lymphoma cells with a monoclonal anti-β chain or anti-α chain reactive antibody plus complement. The negative selection depleted the mutagenized population of cells expressing that particular serologic epitope. The negatively selected cells were then positively immunoselected with another anti-β chain or anti-α chain monoclonal antibody in a flow cytometer. With this procedure cells would be selected that no longer express the serologic epitope used in the initial negative selection step but retained the serologic epitope used in the subsequent positive selection step. The antibodies used in both the negative and positive selection cycles had to be chosen to react to different epitopes on the same class II polypeptide, otherwise chain deletion mutants were usually obtained [59]. The mutant class II-bearing cells were cloned, phenotyped for both antibody and T cell receptor binding site defects and the mutant α or β chain genes were sequenced from cDNA or genomic DNA clones. To be certain that the mutant gene isolated for sequence analysis was responsible for the mutant phenotype of the immunoselected cells, the A^k_β gene from each mutant isolated in our laboratory was subcloned into an expression vector and contransfected with a wild-type A^k_α gene into the Ia negative M12.C3 cells [60]. The resulting Ia positive cells were analyzed serologically to confirm the mutant phenotype.

As shown in table 1, although mutations have been selected in the A^k_β, A^k_α, A^b_α and E^k_β molecules, the most extensive panel of mutants was derived by altering the A^k_β polypeptide (table 1a). This panel of A^k_β mutants was prepared by using different combinations of mAbs from each of the available A^k-serologic specificities to immunoselect unique phenotypes from mutagenized cell populations. Within the panel of A^k_β mutants, each of the major serologic epitopes was altered. DNA sequence analysis of the mutant A^k_β genes revealed that each mutation resulted in a single amino acid substitution and each of the independent substitutions occurred within or near only one of the polymorphic regions in the β_1 domain [60]. The complexity of the serologic epitopes was revealed by the observation that reactivity with several of the monoclonal antibodies was altered by a single substitution at two or more positions. For example, reactivity with mAb 10-2.16 (Ia.17) can be altered by substitution at position 64 (LD3 and G1) or at position 69 (B13). Reactivity with the mAbs of allospecificity Ia.1 was affected by substitution at position 64 (LD3), 69 (B13) or 70 (K5). Furthermore, in three mutants, more than one allodeterminant was altered by the single amino acid substitution. In LD3, Ia.1, Ia.17 and Ia.18 epitopes were altered; in B13, Ia.1 and Ia.17 epitopes were altered; and in

Table 1. Amino acid sequence of different wild-type alleles of A β_1, A α_1 and E β_1 domains as well as the immunoselected mutants from each isotype. Data from ref. [60, 63, 87–90].

Table 1a

```
             10        20        30        40        50        60        70        80        90
k    GNSERHFVHQFQPFCYFTNGTQRIRLVIRYIYNREEYVRFDSDVGEYRAVTELGRPDAEYWNKQ*Y*LERTRAELDTVCRHNYEKTETPTSLRRLE
b    -D------Y--MGE-----------Y-T-----------Y------H-------------------S-PEI-------------------GP--H-------
d    --------V--KGE--Y----------T-----------Y-----------------------S-PEI-------V--A------GP--S-------
f    --------F--KGE-----------S-D---------L-----------------S----Y-----------------------GV----------
q    --------A-LKGE-----------S-N--------W--------------------------S-PEI-------V---------GV--H-------
s    -D------F--KGE-----------S-D---------L----------------------Y--------Q--------------GV--H-------
u    -D-----LV-----------------Y-T---------L----------------------Y-------------------Y---E--V--------

LD3  ---------------------------------------------------------------P--------------------------------
G1   ---------------------------------------------------------------R--------------------------------
K5   ---------------------------------------------------------------------Q--------------------------
F16  ----------------------------------------------------------D-------------------------------------
B13  --------------------------------------------------------------------K---------------------------
```

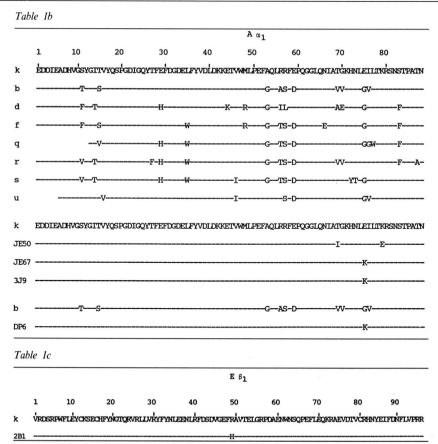

Table 1b

A α_1

```
     1       10        20        30        40        50        60        70        80
k    EDDIEADHVGSYGITVYQSPGDIGQYTFEFDGDELFYVDLDKKETVWMLPEFAQLRRFEPQGGLQNIATGKHNLEILTKRSNSTPATN
b    ----------T---S-------------------------------------G--AS-D---------VV----GV------------
d    ----------F--T--------------H--------------K---R----G--IL-----------AE----G-------F-----
f    ----------F---S-------------------W------------R----G--TS-D------E--------G-------F-----
q                --V-----------H-----W-----------------G--TS-D----------------GGW-----F-----
r    ----------V--T------------F-H-----W-----------------G--TS-D---------VV------------F---A-
s    ----------V--T--------------H-----W----------I------G--TS-D------------YT-G-------------
u         ----------V-----------------------------I----------S-D---------------GV------------

k    EDDIEADHVGSYGITVYQSPGDIGQYTFEFDGDELFYVDLDKKETVWMLPEFAQLRRFEPQGGLQNIATGKHNLEILTKRSNSTPATN
JE50 --------------------------------------------------------------------I---------E---------
JE67 ---------------------------------------------------------------------------K------------
3J9  ---------------------------------------------------------------------------K------------

b    ----------T---S-------------------------------------G--AS-D---------VV----GV------------
DP6  ---------------------------------------------------------------------------K------------
```

Table 1c

E β_1

```
     1       10        20        30        40        50        60        70        80        90
k    VRDSRPWFLEYCKSECHFYNGTQRVRLLVRYFYNLEENLRFDSDVGEFRAVTELGRPDAENWNSQPEFLEQKRAEVDTVCRHNYEIFDNFLVPRR
2B1  ------------------------------------------------H----------------------------------------------
```

F16, Ia.18 and the 40F/40L epitopes were altered. Thus, as with other serologic epitopes, an alloantigenic epitope is created by the interaction of several residues. In addition, these results indicate that serologically distinct epitopes may overlap, perhaps by sharing some contact residues. Alternatively, substitutions in this region may induce conformational alterations at a distant site. However, it seems unlikely that multiple independent substitutions in only this one polymorphic region would be recovered if the major effect of these substitutions was the induction of conformational changes at distant epitopes on the molecule. Thus, these results strongly suggest that this one polymorphic region is the major determinant of alloantigenicity on the A^k_β polypeptide.

In addition to the serologic defects, the A^k_β mutants exhibit a broad spectrum of functional defects when they are used to stimulate a panel of T hybridomas of various specificities. In one study that utilized a combination of antigen and autoreactive T hybridomas, the range of functional phenotypes observed from four class II mutants varied from nearly wild-type (F16 and G1) to nearly completely defective (K5) [59]. However, no pattern of functional reactivities emerged that correlated with either the structural data or the serological phenotypes. In a separate study, the T cell response to hen egg lysozyme (HEL) was measured using a panel of 10 A^k-specific T hybridomas and a panel of 8 serologically selected A^k_β and A^k_α mutant cell lines [61]. Five of the T hybridomas specific for HEL peptide 46–61 exhibited four different patterns of stimulation by the mutant cell lines. These data suggest that multiple determinants can be formed by the association of a 16 residue peptide and the A^k molecule, indirectly indicating the existence of several T cell recognition sites on the A^k molecule.

Four A^k_α mutants (table 1b) have been isolated using an immunoselection protocol and have been characterized serologically, structurally and functionally. Three of the A^k_α mutants have lost the Ia.2 and Ia.19 serologic epitopes but retain the serologic epitopes defined by mAbs 1E9, 3B9 and 4D5 [62]. Two of the α chain mutants, JE67 and 3J9, although produced in different laboratories, contain the identical point mutation resulting in a substitution at position 75 in the α_1 domain [63, 64]. The other A^k_α mutant, JE50, contains nonconservative substitutions at positions 69 and 79 [62]. Although the two different α chain mutants are serologically indistinguishable, they exhibit significant differences when analyzed with a panel of HEL-reactive hybridomas [61, 65]. The JE67 mutant presents HEL to 20 of the 23 T hybridomas tested whereas the mutant JE50 presents HEL to only 6 or the 23 T hybridomas. Thus, although the mutation at position 75 in JE67 eliminates an α chain immunodominant serological epitope (Ia.2 and Ia.19), it has little effect on the presentation of HEL to T cell receptors. One could infer that the lysozyme peptides presented to the T cell receptors are bound to the class II molecule at a site spatially distant from position 75 in the α_1 domain. In addition, position 75, which is accessible to antibodies and therefore likely exposed to the aqueous environment, may not be an important contact point for the association with most of these T cell receptors.

Positions 69 and/or 79 are unlikely to be contact points for peptide binding because at least three different HEL peptides are effectively presented to T hybridomas by JE50 cells [65]. The marked defect in APC capability of the JE50 mutant may result from the failure of T cell receptors to bind to the JE50 class II molecule. The hypothetical model of the class II three-dimensional structure [66], which is based on the results from the class I crystal analysis, predicts that both residues 69 and 79 are exposed to the aqueous environment and point upward where they could contact the T cell antigen receptor.

A single E^k mutant (table 1c) has been produced and shown to contain a point mutation at position 49 in the β_1 domain [67]. Although this mutant class II molecule is defective in the serologic epitope defined by mAb 17.3.3, its ability to function as an antigen presenting cell is unimpaired [68].

In-vitro-Derived Mutants – Genetic Engineering

Two different types of genetically engineered class II mutants have been produced. One type involves the interchange of exons or hemiexons (exon shuffling) from one allele to another and the other involves the production of site specific mutants by introducing residues that are found in other alleles or are novel. In both cases the altered class II genes were expressed after transfection into either murine L cells or B lymphoma cells.

The original reports describing exon shuffled β chain variants showed that the β_1 domain contains all of the immunologically relevant serologic and T cell determinants in the β chain [69, 70]. These studies and others done subsequently failed to find any immunologic functions associated with the α_2/β_2 domain. Germain's laboratory later extended these studies designed to localize the functional regions on the β_1 domain by preparing a series of recombinant genes involving the exchange of halves of the β_1 domain among the *k*, *d* and *b* alleles [71, 72]. The recombinant genes were expressed in L cells. Analysis of the recombinant class II molecules localized the binding sites of five β chain-reactive antibodies to the carboxy-terminal half of the β_1 domain. In contrast, both halves of the β_1 domain were involved in determining T cell recognition sites for a panel of antigen reactive and alloreactive T cell hybridomas. Their analyses also confirmed previous reports that polymorphic residues in both the α and β chains were involved in determining T cell receptor restriction sites [73]. This group also prepared half-exon shuffles between E^k_β and E^b_β β_1 domains and assayed these class II molecules for their ability to present cytochrome *c* to T cell clones [74]. By taking advantage of the limited number of polymorphisms between E^k_β and E^b_β they were able to establish that residue 29 determined the ability of the E^k_β molecule to present cytochrome *c* to the E^k-restricted T cells. When these results were combined with the data on binding of the cytochrome *c* peptide to the E^k_β molecule [1], it was predicted that residue 29 determines the activation of cytochrome-*c*-reactive T cells by controlling the efficiency of peptide binding to E^k_β and E^b_β molecules.

Similarly altered α chain genes have been prepared by shuffling α_1 exon segments between the A^k_α and A^b_α genes [63]. When these genes were expressed in L cells it was found that a series of six anti-A^b_α reactive mAbs mapped to the polymorphic residues at positions 53, 56, 57 and 59. By preparing A^k_α and A^b_α genes with single substitutions at positions 57 and 75, it was determined that the A^k allospecificities Ia.2 and Ia.19 both mapped to the polymorphic difference at residue 75. These results disproved a prediction that Ia.2 would map to position 57 [75]. This prediction was made from sequence comparisons of different alleles and was based on the observation that the Ia.2 determinant is unique to A^k_α and that arg at position 57 is the only residue unique to the A^k_α polypeptide. This example demonstrates that it is not always possible to identify which polymorphic residue determines an antibody binding site solely on the basis of cross-reactivity patterns and sequence data.

When cells expressing these mutant α chain molecules were assayed for their ability to present HEL to a panel of T hybridomas, it was shown that the three different polymorphic regions exerted significantly different effects on the antigen presentation capacity of the class II molecules [65]. Substitution of the polymorphic region between the α chain residues 69 and 76 completely eliminated the presentation of HEL to all T hybridomas assayed. Substitution of the polymorphic region between α chain residues 53 and 59 eliminated the presentation function to approximately half of the T cells and substitution of the polymorphic region between residues 11 to 16 had little, if any, effect. It was predicted from these results that the polymorphic region between α chain residues 69 and 76 will directly contact the HEL peptide while the polymorphic residues between positions 53 and 59 will be primarily involved in contact with the T cell antigen receptor [65].

Although exon shuffling experiments were useful for the initial localization of the functional regions on the class II molecules, the gene segments exchanged were, in general, too large to permit the identification of specific residues comprising either antibody or T cell receptor-binding sites. Cohn et al. [52] constructed three site-directed mutants by introducing *k* allele residues at positions 9, 13 and 65–67 in the A_β^b polypeptide. When the mutant genes were expressed in the Ia negative M12.C3 cells, only the class II molecules that had been altered at positions 65–67 resulted in loss of serologic epitopes characteristic of the A_β^b polypeptide. All three mutants resulted in the loss of at least some allo- or antigen-reactive T cell restriction sites.

In a similar analysis, the effect of each of the three amino acid substitutions in the A_β^{bm12} (positions 67, 70 and 71) were evaluated by introducing each of the bm12 substitutions individually into the A_β^b gene [76]. Of the A_β^b-reactive mAbs that do not react with bm12, all were specific for an epitope determined primarily by the substitution at position 70. In contrast, all three mutant positions significantly altered the antigen presentation function to a panel of T hybridomas. Both of these studies were limited, however, because only the loss of antibody or T cell reactivity was observed. Clearly, the loss of these functions can be due to alteration of contact points or due to conformational alteration of contact points at a spatially distant site on the class II molecule. In addition, only the effects resulting from alteration of a small number of residues in the β_1 domain was evaluated.

We have undertaken an extensive analysis of the structural basis of antibody and T-cell-binding sites on the β_1 domain of the A_β^k and A_β^d polypeptides. We constructed a panel of altered A_β^k genes that encode single or multiple residues of the A_β^d polypeptide at 14 polymorphic positions in the β_1 domain [53] (table 2). The mutant A_β^k polypeptides (designated A_β^{k}*) were expressed in association with either wild-type A_α^k or A_α^d polypeptides after transfection of the genes into the B lymphoma cell line M12.C3. Individual clones expressing comparable levels of the mutant class II molecules were selected and analyzed with a panel of A_β^k- and A_β^d-reactive mAbs as well as with a panel of A_β^k- or A_β^d-alloreactive T cell hybridomas.

The M12.C3 cells are unique recipients for the mutant A_β^{k*} genes in that they constitutively express A_α^d mRNA but no A_β^d mRNA [52]. When the A_β^{k*} gene is cotransfected with pRSV-neo, the neomycin resistant cells express hybrid A_β^{k*} A_α^d molecules on their cell surface (fig. 1). When the A_β^{k*} gene is cotransfected with a wild-type A_α^k gene and pRSV-veo, the neomycin resistant cells primarily express A_β^{k*} A_α^k molecules on their cell surface because A_β^k polypeptides preferentially associate with A_α^k polypeptides rather than A_α^d polypeptides. The selective expression of either A_β^{k*} A_α^k molecules or A_β^{k*} A_α^d molecules is very useful to elucidate the interactions of A_β and A_α polymorphic residues in mAb binding, T_R binding and in determining the preferential chain association phenomena.

Table 2. Mutants of the murine I–A β_1 domain.

```
MUTANTS OF THE MURINE I-A β1 DOMAIN

                         10         20         30         40         50         60         70         80         90
                         I          I          I          I          I          I          I          I          I
k wt            GNSERHFVHQ FQPFCTFTNG TQRIRLVIRY IYNREEYVRF DSDVGEYRAV TELGRPDAEY WNKQ Y LER TRAELDTVCR HNYEKTETPT SLRRLE

d wt            --------V- -KGE--Y--- -------T-- ---------Y ---------- ---------- --S-PEI--- ----V--A-- ----GP--S- ------

Mutants with single changes

TF.9            --------V- ---------- ---------- ---------- ---------- ---------- ---- - --- ---------- ---------- ------
TF.12           ---------- -K-------- ---------- ---------- ---------- ---------- ---- - --- ---------- ---------- ------
TF.13           ---------- --G------- ---------- ---------- ---------- ---------- ---------- ---------- ---------- ------
TF.14           ---------- ---E------ ---------- ---------- ---------- ---------- ---- - --- ---------- ---------- ------
TF.17           ---------- ------Y--- ---------- ---------- ---------- ---------- ---- - --- ---------- ---------- ------
TF.21           ---------- ---------- A--------- ---------- ---------- ---------- ---- - --- ---------- ---------- ------
TF.28           ---------- ---------- -------T-- ---------- ---------- ---------- ---- - --- ---------- ---------- ------
TF.40           ---------- ---------- ---------- ---------Y ---------- ---------- ---- - --- ---------- ---------- ------
TF.63           ---------- ---------- ---------- ---------- ---------- ---------- --S- - --- ---------- ---------- ------
TF.65           ---------- ---------- ---------- ---------- ---------- ---------- ----PEI--- ---------- ---------- ------
TF.75           ---------- ---------- ---------- ---------- ---------- ---------- ---- - --- ----V----- ---------- ------
TF.78           ---------- ---------- ---------- ---------- ---------- ---------- ---- - --- -------A-- ---------- ------
TF.85           ---------- ---------- ---------- ---------- ---------- ---------- ---- - --- ---------- ----G----- ------
TF.86           ---------- ---------- ---------- ---------- ---------- ---------- ---- - --- ---------- -----P---- ------
TF.89           ---------- ---------- ---------- ---------- ---------- ---------- ---- - --- ---------- --------S- ------

Mutants with regional changes

TF.A            --------V- -KGE--Y--- ---------- ---------- ---------- ---------- ---- - --- ---------- ---------- ------
TF.B            ---------- ---------- ---------- ---------- ---------- ---------- --S-PEI--- ---------- ---------- ------
TF.C            ---------- ---------- ---------- ---------- ---------- ---------- ---- - --- ----V--A-- ---------- ------
TF.D            ---------- ---------- ---------- ---------- ---------- ---------- ---------- ---------- ----GP--S- ------

TF.AB           --------V- -KGE--Y--- ---------- ---------- ---------- ---------- --S-PEI--- ---------- ---------- ------
TF.AC           --------V- -KGE--Y--- ---------- ---------- ---------- ---------- ---- - --- ----V--A-- ---------- ------
TF.AD           --------V- -KGE--Y--- ---------- ---------- ---------- ---------- ---- - --- ---------- ----GP--S- ------
TF.CD           ---------- ---------- ---------- ---------- ---------- ---------- ---- - --- ----V--A-- ----GP--S- ------

TF.ACD          --------V- -KGE--Y--- ---------- ---------- ---------- ---------- ---- - --- ----V--A-- ----GP--S- ------
TF.BCD          ---------- ---------- ---------- ---------- ---------- ---------- --S-PEI--- ----V--A-- ----GP--S- ------
TF.ABC          --------V- -KGE--Y--- ---------- ---------- ---------- ---------- --S-PEI--- ----V--A-- ---------- ------
```

A panel of mAbs that exhibits a spectrum of different A_β^k reactivities was used to assay for loss of A_β^k serologic epitopes [53]. Among the mutant A_β^{k*} molecules that contained single *d* allele substitutions, only those mutants with substitutions at positions 63 or 65–67 showed any detectable loss of antibody binding (table 3). The substitution of the d-allele serine at position 62 eliminated the binding of antibody 40F,

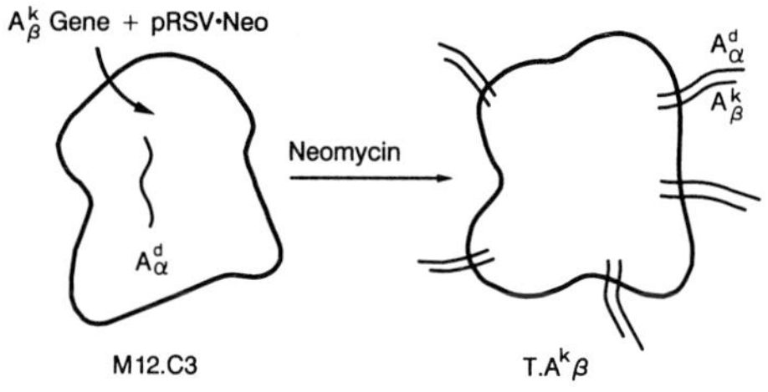

a

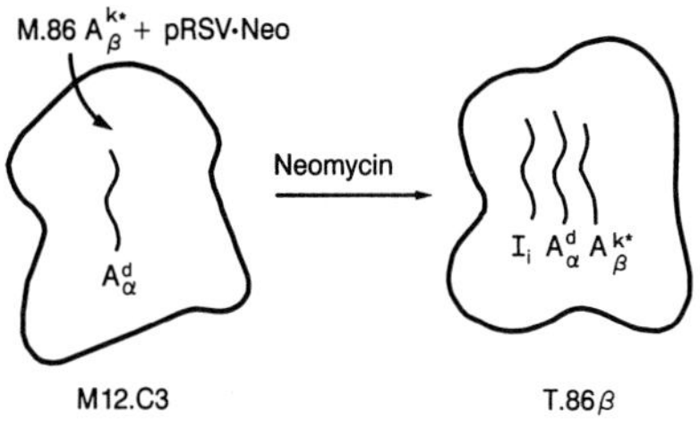

b

Fig. 1. Transfection of A^{k*}_β genes into M12.C3 cells. M12.C3 cells contain endogenous A^d_α mRNA but no A^d_β mRNA. Mutant A^{k*}_β genes, constructed by site-directed mutagenesis, are expressed with high efficiency in these cells. The A^{k*}_β genes are cotransfected by electroporation with the neomycin selection marker (pRSV-neo) into M12.C3 cells. As shown in *a*, transfected, neomycin resistant cells express on their surface high levels of A^{k*}_β A^d_α molecules. In *b*, when the A^{k*}_β gene is cotransfected with the wild-type A^k_α gene and pRSV-neo the transfected, neomycin resistant cells primarily express A^{k*}_β A^k_α molecules on their surface. The hybrid molecules (A^{k*}_β A^d_β) are expressed at low levels on the cell surface due to the preferential association of A^k_β for A^k_α polypeptides.

whereas the three-for-one residue insertion at positions 65–67 eliminated the binding of the antibodies that define the allospecificities Ia.1, Ia.17 and Ia.18. When mutant class II molecules containing multiple (entire polymorphic region) *d* allele substitutions were tested with the same mAbs, only those mutants expressing *d* allele residues in region ‘B’ (residues 63 and 65–67) exhibited loss of the serological epitopes (table 4). In addition, the mutant containing *d* allele residues in nearly the entire β_1 domain (T.ACD) while maintaining *k* allele residues in region ‘B’, showed wild-type levels of binding of all A^k_β-reactive mAbs. Together, these results, which show that the A^k_β serologic epitopes are maintained despite substitution of all A^d_β polymorphic residues in the β_1 domain outside of

Table 3. Cytofluorometric analysis of M12.C3 cell lines transfected with mutant A_β^k genes which encode residues of the A_β^d polypeptide at single positions in the β_1 domain[1]

Monoclonal antibodies	Cell lines															
	T.Neo[2]	T.A^{k}[3]	T9	T12	T13	T14	T17	T28	T40	T63	T65–67	T75	T78	T85	T86	T89
39B	–	+++	+++	+++	+++	++	+++	+++	+++	+++	–	+++	+++	++	++	+++
39E	–	+++	+++	+++	+++	++	++	+++	+++	+++	–	+++	+++	+++	+++	+++
40M	–	+++	+++	+++	+++	++	+++	+++	+++	+++	–	+++	+++	+++	+++	+++
10.2–16	–	+++	+++	+++	+++	++	++	+++	++	+++	–	+++	+++	+++	++	+++
11–3.25	–	+++	+++	+++	+++	+++	+++	+++	+++	+++	–	+++	+++	+++	+++	+++
4–2.1	–	+++	+++	+++	+++	++	++	+++	++	+++	–	+++	+++	+++	+++	+++
4–2.3	–	+++	+++	+++	++	++	+++	+++	+++	+++	–	N.D.	+++	++	+++	+++
40F	–	+++	+++	+++	+++	++	+++	+++	+++	–	+++	+++	+++	+++	+++	+++
+++	++	+	++	+++	+++	+++	+++	+++	+++	+++	+++	+++	+++			
K24–199[5]	–	+	–	++	+	–	–	–	–	+	–	–	–	–	–	–

[1] The transfected cell lines were divided into four categories based upon levels of antibody binding relative to the wild-type TA3 cell line. The peak fluorescence channel difference between cells stained with the negative antibody and cells stained with the antibody in question was divided through the peak channel difference obtained for the TA3 cell line with the same antibodies in the same experiment and then multiplied by 100. – = Values less than 5%; + = values 5–25%; ++ = values 26–75%; +++ = values more than 75%. Data from Buerstedde et al. [53].

[2] Cell line transfected only with the neomycin resistance gene.

[3] Cell line transfected with the wild-type A_α^k and A_β^k gene.

[4] 39J recognizes the A_α^k polypeptide.

[5] K24–199 recognizes the A_α^d polypeptide.

Table 4. Cytofluorometric analysis of M12.C3 cell lines transfected with mutant A_β^k genes which encode single or multiple regions of the A_β^d polypeptide in the β_1 domain[1]

Monoclonal antibodies	Cell lines						
	T.A.	T.B.	T.C.	T.D.	T.ABC	T.ACD	T.BCD
39B	+++	–	+++	+++	–	+++	–
39E	+++	–	+++	+++	–	+++	–
40M	+++	–	+++	+++	–	+++	–
10.2–16	+++	–	+++	+++	–	+++	–
11–3.25	+++	–	+++	+++	–	+++	–
4–2.3	+++	–	+++	+++	–	+++	–
4–2.3	+++	–	+++	+++	–	+++	–
40F	+++	–	+++	+++	–	+++	–
39J[2]	–	+++	+++	+++	–	–	+++
K24–199[3]	+++	+	–	–	+++	+++	–

[1] The TA3 cell line was used as a standard (see under table 3). Data from Buerstedde et al. [53].
[2] 39J recognizes the A_α^k polypeptide.
[3] K24–199 recognizes the A_α^d polypeptide.

region 'B', clearly demonstrate serologic immunodominance of region 'B' of the A^k_β polypeptide.

Theoretically, serologic epitopes can be lost in these class II mutants by altering residues in the contact site or by introducing at distant sites substitutions that change the conformation of the serologic epitope. However, the gain of a serologic epitope likely will occur only when the appropriate antibody contact residues are restored. We, therefore, tested a panel of eight A^d_β-reactive mAbs for binding to the panel of A^{k*}_β mutants to determine if serologic epitopes characteristic of the *d* allele were introduced into the A^k_β polypeptide [53]. As shown in table 5, three of the A^d_β-reactive antibodies reacted to mutant A^{k*}_β molecules containing *d* allele residues at positions 65–67. Another antibody reacted to the A^{k*}_β mutant with *d* allele residues at positions 63 and 65–67, another reacted with the A^{k*}_β mutant with *d* allele residues at either positons 63 or 40, and yet another reacted with the A^{k*}_β mutant containing a single *d* allele residue at position 40. The binding site of another mAb mapped to a complex of *d* allele residues in regions 'B' and 'C'. Thus, the introduction of *d* allele residues at positions 40, 63 and/or 65–67 resulted in the binding of most A^d_β-reactive mAbs. The observed gain of the A^d_β serologic epitopes parallels the observed cross-reactivity patterns of these antibodies on known class II alelles. For example, antibodies that react with the T.40 mutant cross-react on the alleles *b*, *d*, *r* and *v*, but not on alleles *f*, *k*, *q*, *s*, *u* and *p*. Alleles *b* and *d* both have tyr at position 40 while alleles *f*, *k*, *q*, *s*, and *u* have a phe at position 40. The other alleles (*p*, *r*, *v*) have not been sequenced. These results suggest that these serologic epitopes are determined primarily by one polymorphic residue or a limited number of polymorphic residues on each cross-reacting allele. Thus, results from analyses of both the immunoselected class II mutants and the site directed mutants are concordant and demonstrate that there is a serologically immunodominant site in the A^k_β and A^d_β polypeptide near positions 60–70.

This analysis of the A^{k*}_β site-directed class II mutants is, however, limited to identifying polymorphic residues that are involved in determining the serologic epitopes. It is clear from the analysis of the immunoselected mutants that different combinations of nonpolymorphic residues also contribute to the composition of the different epitopes. Until the complete three-dimensional crystal structure is solved, it will be very difficult to obtain additional unambiguous information concerning the identification of the nonpolymorphic residues that determine the serologic epitopes. Although it is possible to produce additional β chain mutants with substitutions at the nonpolymorphic residues, it is very difficult to determine if the substitution directly causes the loss of a serologic epitope or if the substitution induces a conformational change that alters a spatially distant

Table 5. Cytofluorometric analysis of mutant A^k_β bearing cell lines with antibodies reactive to A^d_β

Monoclonal antibodies	Cell lines														
	T.A^{k1}	T.A$^{k2}_\beta$	T.A$^{d/k3}$	T28	T40	T40β^4	T63	T65	T.A	T.B	T.C	T.D	T.ABC	T.ACD	T.BCD
25–9–17S	–	–	+++	–	–	–	–	++	–	+++	–	–	+++	–	+++
34–5–3S	–	–	+++	–	–	–	–	++	–	+++	–	–	+++	–	+++
Y-237	–	–	+++	–	–	–	–	+	–	++	–	–	++	–	+
Y-276	–	–	+++	–	–	–	–	–	–	+++	–	–	+++	–	+++
Y-219	–	–	+++	–	+	++	–	–	–	–	–	–	–	–	–
Y-270	–	–	+++	–	+	–	–	–	–	–	–	–	–	–	–
Y-212	–	–	+++	–	+	++	+++	–	–	++	–	–	+	–	+
MKD	–	–	+++	–	–	–	–	–	–	–	–	–	++	–	++

The TA3 cell line was used as a standard (see under table 3). Data from Buerstedde et al. [53].
[1] Cell line transfected with the wild-type A^k_α and A^k_β gene.
[2] Cell line transfected only with the wild-type A^k_β gene.
[3] Cell line transfected with an A^k_β gene construct in which the second exon was derived from the A^d_β gene.
[4] Cell line transfected only with the M40 A^k_β gene.

epitope. Since it is difficult, at best, to obtain chemical quantities of class II molecules sufficient for optical conformational analyses, it is unlikely that this problem will be overcome in the near future.

This panel of class II mutants has been analyzed for its ability to stimulate a panel of A^k_β- and A^d_β-alloreactive T cell hybridomas [77]. As shown in table 5, we have been able to map to specific β chain polymorphic residues the T cell binding sites for a number of the T hybridomas. The antigen receptors on the T hybridomas 59.16 and 22.1 recognize *k* allele polymorphic residues in the β_1 domain as well as A^k_α polymorphic residues. In contrast the antigen receptors on the T hybridoma 98.11 recognize *k* allele polymorphic residues in the β_1 domain but do not discriminate A^k_α from A^d_α polymorphic residues. When these three A^k-reactive T hybridomas were assayed for their response to different class II mutant molecules, the hybridomas 59.16 and 22.1 responded to the class II mutant T.BCD, which contains *d* allele residues in the entire C-terminal half of the β_1 domain. Both hybridomas also reacted to mutants T.28 and T.40. These results suggest that the antigen receptors on these two T hybridomas recognize β chain residues within the polymorphic region 'A' (residues 9–17). Since the mutant A^{k*}_β polypeptide containing *d* allele residues in region 'A' cannot be expressed in association with the A^k_α polypeptide, we cannot directly assess if the mutant T.A A^{k*}_β A^k_α molecule will stimulate these two T hybridomas. However, when we dissected the potential contribution of the 'A' region by testing class II molecules consisting of a wild-type A^k_α polypeptide and a mutant A^{k*}_β polypeptide containing single *d* allele residues at either position 9, 12, 13, 14, or 17 we found that the T hybridoma 22.1 is not stimulated by any of the mutants while T hybridoma 59.16 is not stimulated by mutants 12, 13 or 14. Thus, the specificities of these two A^k-reactive T hybridomas map to two similar sites on the β_1 domain. In contrast, T hybridoma 98.11 is stimulated at wild-type levels by the mutant T.A A^k_β A^d_α. Since 98.11 is not stimulated by A^{k*}_β mutants with *d* allele substitutions in any of the three regions 'B', 'C' or 'D', the antigen receptors on this hybridoma appear to recognize a complex epitope determined by multiple *k* allele polymorphic residues in regions 'B', 'C' and 'D'.

Mapping studies that utilize loss of functional epitopes must be interpreted with caution. Conformational alterations at spatially distant sites may be introduced by the mutations and such conformational alterations can be very difficult to detect without direct physiochemical measurements. An alternative to measuring the mutation-induced loss of *k* allele allospecificities is to assay for the gain of *d* allele allospecificities in the mutants. As previously discussed, it is likely that the gain of the allospecificity will be due directly to the structural alterations introduced by the *d* allele polymorphic residues. In addition, the identification of an epitope gain in the A_{β}^{k*} mutants suggests that the overall class II structure is intact in the mutant and any observed loss of '*k*' reactivity is not due to gross structural abnormalities.

When three A^{d}-reactive T hybridomas were assayed on the panel of A_{β}^{k*} mutants, each of the T cells was stimulated by class II molecules comprised of wild-type A_{α}^{d} polypeptides associated with a A_{β}^{k*} molecule containing *d* allele residues throughout the entire β_1 domain (β1D.β) (table 5). The T cell receptor epitopes mapped to *d* allele residues in the β_1 domain because the T hybridomas did not respond to class II molecules containing A_{β}^{k} polypeptides. We could not evaluate the α chain contribution of the T cell specificity because the A_{α}^{k} polypeptide does not associate with the A_{β}^{d} polypeptide. Each of the T hybridomas exhibited a distinctive reactivity pattern. T hybridoma DG11 is stimulated at wild-type levels by class II molecules consisting of a wild-type A_{α}^{d} polypeptide and a T.B A_{β}^{k*} polypeptide. The T cells were also stimulated, albeit less efficiently, with the T.65–67 A_{β}^{k*} A_{α}^{d} molecule. Polymorphic residues in region 'B' (63 and 65–67) were previously shown to be directly responsible for determining the loss of A_{β}^{k}-reactive serologic epitopes and the gain of A_{β}^{d}-reactive serologic epitopes [53]. Thus, the DG11 antigen receptor recognizes an epitope comprised, in part, of the same polymorphic residues that comprise the immunodominant β chain serologic epitope. Whether the same non-polymorphic residues are involved in determining both the serologic and T cell epitopes cannot be evaluated with this type of mutant analysis. The A^{d}-reactive T hybridoma IC4 reacts at wild-type response levels to a class II molecule comprised of a wild-type A_{α}^{d} molecule and a T.AD A_{β}^{k*} polypeptide. Since the substitution of *d* allele residues in region 'A' alone or region 'D' alone is not sufficient to produce a functional epitope for these T cell receptors, the receptors must recognize a complex epitope comprised of multiple polymorphic residues that are widely separated in the β_1 domain primary sequence. We have been unable to map the epitope recognized by the receptors on the T hybridoma D1G1. This receptor may recognize a complex epitope comprised of either a large number of polymorphic residues or some combination of polymorphic residues not represented in this panel of A_{β}^{k*} mutants.

The results of these analyses demonstrate that some T cell receptors bind to the same β_1 domain polymorphic residues as do antibodies. However, at least in this limited sample of alloreactive T cell hybridomas, most of the T cells were stimulated by polymorphic residues in regions of the β_1 domain that are distinct from the β chain serologically immunodominant region. Such results are consistent with a variety of functional analyses indicating that antibodies and T cell receptors recognize different regions on the class II molecule [73]. In the final section of this review, these results will be evaluated in the context of the hypothetical three-dimensional structural model of the class II molecule.

Class II Mutants – Regulation of Cell Surface Expression

In 1980, Kimoto and Fathman [78] demonstrated that T cell receptors could be restricted to either parental (e.g. A^k_β A^k_α, A^b_β A^b_α) class II molecules or hybrid (e.g. A^k_β A^b_α, A^b_β A^k_α) molecules in the F_1 ($k \times b$) animal. These authors suggested that the ability to make use of hybrid class II molecules as restriction elements would expand the immunologic response capacity of a heterozygous animal over that of a homozygous one. This potential heterozygote selective advantage could provide at least one explanation for the high level of natural heterozygosity at these MHC loci. However, several reports have documented that not all A and E isotype hybrid class II molecules are expressed with equal efficiency [79–82]. For example, Germain et al. [82] reported that A^d_β A^k_α molecules are not expressed and A^k_β A^d_α molecules are expressed at very low levels in L cells. Using hemi-exon shuffled mutants, Braunstein and Germain [72] demonstrated that the polymorphic residues in the N-terminal half of the β chain were responsible for controlling the efficiency of this $k \times d$ heterodimer expression. We have used our panel of A^{k*}_β mutants to identify the β_1 domain residues responsible for the preferential cell surface expression of the A^k_β polypeptide with either the A^k_α polypeptide or the A^d_α polypeptide [37]. We observed that *d* allele substitutions at positions 12 and 13 are primarily responsible for controlling the expression of A^d_β A^k_α molecules. Mutant T.12 and T.13 A^{k*}_β polypeptides exhibited altered association with A^k_α polypeptides and the substitution of *d* allele residues in the entire region 'A' (residues 9, 12, 13, 14 and 17) of the A^{k*}_β polypeptide completely inhibited association with the A^k_α polypeptide. This expression defect cannot be overcome by the substitution of additional *d* allele residues at other positions in the β_1 domain [37]. Presumably, the side chains of these β chains polymorphic residues interact with the side chains of polymorphic residues on the α chain in a manner that affects heterodimer formation.

In contrast to results reported by Germain et al. [82], we have observed that A^k_β A^d_α hybrid molecules are expressed at high levels in the B lymphoma M12.C3 cells as long as the cells do not concurrently express the A^k_α polypeptide [53]. In the absence of the A^k_α polypeptide, the A^k_β and A^d_α polypeptides associate effectively and are expressed on the cell surface at high levels. However, there is a preferential association of the A^k_β and A^k_α polypeptides that effectively prevents most of the association of the A^k_β A^d_α molecules in the normal heterozygous situation. One could use these

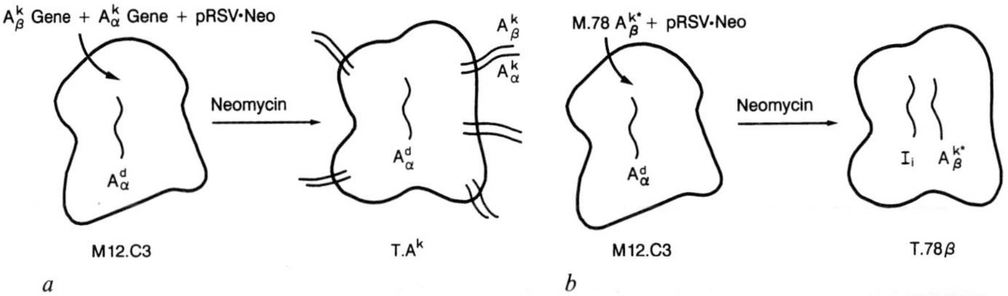

Fig. 2. Expression of M.86 A_β^{k*} and M.78 A_β^{k*} genes in M12.C3 cells. *a* M.86 A_β^{k*} genes cotransfected with the neomycin selection marker (pRSV-neo) into M12.C3 cells express little or no T.86 A_β^{k*} A_α^d molecules on their cell surface but they do express T.86 A_β^{k*} A_α^d I_i complexes intracellularly. M12.C3 cells cotransfected with M.86 A_β^{k*} genes, wild-type A_α^k genes and pRSV-neo, express high levels of M.86 A_β^{k*} A_α^k molecules on their cell surface [37]. *b* M.78 A_β^{k*} genes cotransfected with pRSV-neo into M12.C3 cells express no T.78 A_β^{k*} A_α^d molecules on their cell surface but do express T.78 A_β^{k*} I_i complexes intracellularly. When M.78 A_β^{k*} genes are cotransfected with wild-type A_α^k genes and pRSV-neo, the neomycin resistant cells express high levels of T.78 A_β^{k*} A_α^k molecules on their surface.

observations to question the biological significance of hybrid class II molecules in T cell restriction. Although it is clear that $A^k \times A^b$ hybrids form unique T cell determinants, there are multiple examples in within both A and E isotypes where the hybrid molecules do not appear to associate effectively. If these hybrid molecules provided a significant selection advantage by providing additional restriction elements for antigen specific immune responses then one would expect that the observed preferential chain association would be selected against in the population.

We have also identified mutations in the C-terminal end of the β_1 domain that either completely inhibit A_β^{k*} A_α^d expression or result in the expression of the A_β^{k*} A_α^d molecule primarily in an intracellular compartment [37]. The substitution of a single *d* allele residue at position 86 in the A_β^{k*} polypeptide results in the expression of very low levels of the mutant T.86 A_β^{k*} A_α^d polypeptide on the cell surface (fig. 2). Analysis of the T.86 Ia immunoprecipitates on two-dimensional gels demonstrated that the T.86 A_β^{k*}, A_α^d and I_i polypeptides are present in the immune complex and the polypeptides are present in the highly glycosylated, mature forms. These results suggest that these molecules are not being transported properly to the cell surface but, since they are normally glycosylated, they are at least transported to the trans cisternae of the Golgi. The I_i polypeptide, which has been hypothesized to be involved in regulating the intracytoplasmic transport of class II molecules, is apparently associated normally with the T.86 Ia molecule and is not likely responsible for the altered cell surface expression. It is possible that the T.86 substitution has induced a conformational alteration in the class II structure that results in abnormal rates of degradation of the T.86 A_β^{k*} A_α^d molecule. However, this potential conformational alteration does not result in an alteration of antibody binding to the T.86 A_β^{k*} mutant. It also should be noted that the T.86 A_β^{k*} A_α^k molecule is expressed on the cell surface at wild-type levels. Thus, the substitution of a single *d* allele residue at position 86 in the A_β^{k*} polypeptide alters the expression of the class II molecule in an allele specific manner. In addition, the substitution of additional *d* allele residues in the T.86 A_β^{k*} β_1 domain restores the expression of the T.86 A_β^{k*} A_α^d molecule on the cell surface (e.g. T.ACD and T.BCD). Thus, it is unlikely that, as previously hypothesized for other immunoselected class II mutants that exhibit a similar expression phenotype [83], the T.86 substitution alters a putative transport signal encoded in the primary sequence of the β_1 domain.

The substitution of a single *d* allele residue at position 78 in the β_1 domain also results in inhibition of expression of the T.78 A_β^{k*} A_α^d molecule, but wild-type levels of expression are maintained when the T.78 A_β^{k*} polypeptide associates with the A_α^k polypeptide. Biochemical analysis of the T.78 A_β^{k*} A_α^d immunoprecipitates demonstrated that the T.78 A_β^{k*} polypeptide and the A_α^d polypeptide do not associate intracellularly. Interestingly, the T.78 A_β^{k*} polypeptide does associate with the I_i polypeptide [37]. Since neither polypeptide contains complex oligosaccharides, it is likely that this T.78 A_β^{k*} I_i complex is located in the endoplasmic reticulum. Although little is known about the requirements for I_i polypeptide association with the α/β complex, these results demonstrate that the I_i polypeptide is capable of associating with the A_β polypeptide in the absence of the A_α polypeptide.

As previously shown with the T.86 mutant, the T.78 A_β^{k*} A_α^d expression phenotype can be corrected if additional *d* allele residues are substituted in the T.78 A_β^{k*} β_1 domain. Although neither T.C nor T.CD A_β^{k*} A_α^d molecules are expressed, T.AC, T.ACD and T.BCD A_β^{k*} A_α^d molecules are expressed at wild-type levels. The side chain of residue 78 may provide a critical interaction with A_α^d polymorphic residues to maintain α/β association. Sequence comparisons of murine and human β chain genes have shown that the region around residue 78 is conserved evolutionarily. Thus, there may be significant structural constraints on the potential substitutions that can occur in this region of the β_1 domain.

Structure-Function Models

Bjorkman et al. [25, 26] have reported the three-dimensional structure of the human class I histocompatibility antigen, A2. The α_1 and α_2 domains interact to form the most external domain and the α_3 domain and β_2 microglobulin interact to form the domain adjacent to the plasma membrane. Residues in the α_1 and α_2 domains form a platform comprised of an eight stranded β-pleated sheet topped by two α helices. The two α helices and the β sheet structure together form a groove that is hypothesized to be the site responsible for binding peptide antigens. Brown et al. [66] have recently used this class I crystal structure to develop a model of the three-dimensional structure of class II molecules. In this model, the class II α_1 region replaces the class I α_1 region and the class II β_1 region replaces the class I α_2 region. It should be emphasized that this is a hypothetical model, which very likely will require revision as additional information about the interactions of the α and β chain residues become available. This caveat is particularly relevant with regard to positioning of the α chain residues. These class II residues were aligned in the model on the basis of matching class I and class II polymorphic residues because of the lack of statistically significant pairwise homology between class I α_1 residues and class II α_1 residues. Despite these reservations the model provides a valuable tool to begin to understand where different α and β residues may be located in the three-dimensional structure of the class II molecule.

Figures 3 and 4 depict a model of the predicted structure of the class II molecule. Although this model is adapted largely from Brown's report, additional modifications have been introduced based on secondary structure predictions made with algorithms developed by Chou and Fasman [84]. In this model, region 'A' of the β_1 domain (residues 9–17) is predicted to be located in the bottom of the groove between the two α helices. Since region 'A' is predicted to be located in the middle of a β strand adjacent to a β strand comprised of the amino-terminal region of the α chain, the introduction of *d* allele residues into region 'A' of the A_β^{k*} polypeptide could affect the interaction of these two β strands. The observation that the residues controlling the preferential chain association phenomena map to region 'A' indicates that the interaction of these two β strands is crucial for the stabilization of the A_β^{k*} A_α^d complex. Substitution of residues in this region could also have a major effect on antigen binding. Since this region is located at the bottom of the putative antigen binding site, substitutions in region 'A' could directly alter the antigen contact site. Alternatively, the conformation of the antigen-binding site could be altered indirectly if substitutions in region 'A' affected the interaction with the α chain polymorphic residues.

Region 'B' (residues 63–67) of the A_β^{k*} polypeptide is predicted to be located in the turn that joins two α helices on the top of the platform comprised of the β-pleated sheet. The side chains of residues 63, 65, 66 and 67 are likely exposed to the aqueous environment since they comprise the

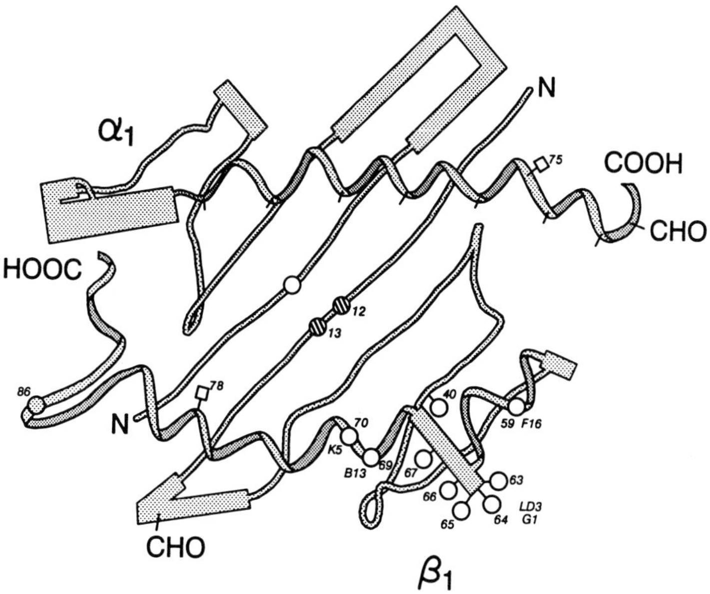

Fig. 3. Location of β chain mutations in the hypothetical model of the class II α_1/β_1 domain. The immunoselected A_β^k mutants F16, LD3, G1, B13 and K5 have been shown to contain point mutations at positions 59, 64, 64, 69 and 70, respectively in the β_1 domain. These positions are located in a region spatially adjacent to the polymorphic residues 40, 63 and 65–67, which have been shown to comprise the serologically immunodominant site in the A_β^k and A_β^d polypeptides. Substitution of *d* allele residues at position 78 or 86 in the A_β^{k*} polypeptide results in expression variants when the A_β^{k*} polypeptide associates with the A_β^d polypeptide. The model is modified from Brown et al. [66]. Regions in shown boxes did not have sufficient homology with the HLA A2 sequence to be able to predict the location of the polypeptide backbone [66].

immunodominant serologic determinant of the β_1 domain. Residue 40 was predicted from the serologic analysis of the A_β^{k*} mutants to be spatially adjacent to residue 63 because both residues were shown to comprise an important determinant for certain *d* allele reactive mAbs. The model is consistent with this prediction. Residue 40 appears to be located on a β strand just under the turn comprised of residues 63–67 (fig. 3). Results from analyses of the immunoselected mutants demonstrate that substitution of adjacent nonpolymorphic residues significantly alters different sets of serologic epitopes. However, it is difficult to determine if these substitutions directly or indirectly affect these serologic epitopes.

Region ‘C’ (residues 75 and 78) is predicted to be located on the α helix that constitutes one side of the putative antigen-binding site. Our mapping data indicate that the mAb MKD6 recognizes an epitope com-

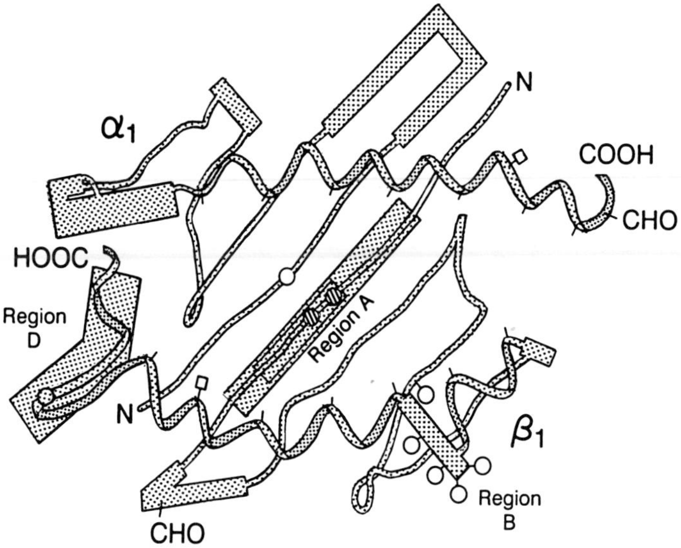

Fig. 4. Location of the polymorphic residues responsible for allospecific T cell receptor binding. Polymorphic residues in region B comprise the immunodominant serologic epitope and the binding site for the A^d-reactive T hybridoma, DG11. Polymorphic residues in region A or region A plus region D are responsible for binding the A^k-reactive T hybridomas 59.16, 22.1 and 98.11. Model is modified from Brown et al. [66].

prised of polymorphic residues in regions 'B' and 'C' [53]. The model is not consistent with these results because it predicts that the two polymorphic residues in region 'C' should project inward into the putative antigen binding site and may not be readily accessible to antibody. We also demonstrated that the substitution of a single *d* allele residue at position 78 disrupts α/β chain association [37]. The substitution of an Ala for Val at 78 is a relatively conservative substitution and would not be expected to significantly alter the charge or relative hydrophobicity of this region. The side chain of this *d* allele residue at position 78 may either directly disrupt a requisite interaction with an α chain polymorphic residue or may alter the conformation of the class II molecule such that an α chain polymorphic residue interaction necessary for proper chain association is disrupted. The class II model predicts that the side chain of residue 78 should not be in direct contact with any α chain polymorphic residue. Thus, the model does not suggest a testable hypothesis for identifying the structural alteration induced by the *d* allele substitution at position 78. Experiments are in progress to determine which *k* allele α chain polymorphic residues will complement the observed expression defect introduced by the substitution at position 78 in the A_β^{k*} sequence.

Region 'D' (residues 85, 86 and 89) is located in a region of the β_1 domain that did not have sufficient homology with the class I sequence to permit modeling of the structure [66]. However, secondary structure predictions suggest that these three residues are located in a turn between the α helix comprised of residues 70–82 and another short helix comprised of residues 92–96. The class I crystal structure suggests that the latter α helix is nearly perpendicular to the former helix and is part of a connecting element linking the β_1 and β_2 domains. We have demonstrated that the substitution of a single *d* allele residue at position 86 alters the cell surface expression of the T.86 A_β^{k*} A_α^d molecule but does not alter expression of the T.86 A_β^{k*} A_α^k molecule [37]. It is possible that the pro for thr substitution significantly alters the secondary structure of the β chain in this turn, which could change how one or both helices interact with α chain polymorphic residues. Such an alteration could destabilize the conformation of the molecule and result in a rapid degradation of the improperly folded molecule. This putative conformational alteration is likely a localized change because our antibody binding studies do not detect any alteration in the T.86 A_β^{k*} serologic epitopes. The class I crystal structure suggests that residue 86 may be adjacent to the α chain polymorphic residues near position 50. Experiments are in progress to determine if the substitution of A_α^d polymorphic residues with *k* allele residues will complement the expression defect induced by the substitution at position 86 in the A_β^{k*} sequence.

The positions we have identified as contributing to T cell antigen receptor binding sites are predicted to be located in at least two distinct areas of the class II molecule (fig. 4). The polymorphic residues that map to the DG11 T hybridoma site are the same residues identified as comprising the A_β^k serologic immunodominant site. In the class II model, these residues [65–67] are predicted to be located on the exterior of the β_1 domain [66]. In contrast, the polymorphic residues in region 'A' (residues 9–17) have been identified as components of the T cell receptor epitopes for three of the six T hybridomas assayed. The epitope for each of these three hybridomas maps to different polymorphic residues in region 'A' or to polymorphic residues in 'A' plus residues in region 'D'. As described previously, region 'A' is located at the bottom of the putative antigen binding site. Region 'A' and 'D' polymorphic residues are located in spatially distant sites in both the primary sequence and in the predicted three-dimensional model (fig. 4). Although these polymorphic residues are predicted to be located sufficiently close together to be within the limits of an antibody-combining site (assuming a T cell receptor combining site is of comparable size), whether these residues are positioned such that they can be contact sites for a T cell receptor is a matter of speculation.

It has been hypothesized that the ligand recognized by alloreactive T cell receptors is comprised of a combination of foreign class II residues and residues of a processed peptide located in the class II antigen-binding site [85]. A recent study demonstrating that $V\beta17a^+$ alloreactive T cells are reactive to E^+ B cells but not to E^+ macrophages or fibroblasts expressing the transfected E genes is consistent with this theory [86]. Our mapping studies completed to date do not enable us to differentiate experimentally between the two possibilities. The observation that the T cell epitopes we have identified map to at least two distinct regions in the class II molecule could indicate that both types of ligands may exist. For example, T cell receptor epitopes that map to the bottom of the putative antigen-binding site (region 'A') may be ligands that are comprised of some combination of residues from a processed peptide and the foreign class II molecule. If this is correct then our mapping studies may have identified the residues involved in binding a processed peptide rather than the residues that contact the T cell receptor. If our limited analysis is representative of the normal T cell repertoire, then the majority of the alloreactive T cells will bind to a similar complex ligand. In contrast, T cell receptor epitopes that map to the same polymorphic residues that comprise the β chain immunodominant serologic epitope may be ligands that are made up of only foreign class II residues. Functional analyses of the immunoselected β chain mutants, however, demonstrated that substitutions in the polymorphic region 'B' can significantly alter the ability of class II molecules to function as restriction elements for antigen-reactive T cells. Additional studies are needed to determine if these substitutions alter the T cell receptor-binding site or the residues that contact the processed peptide. Although we have identified two potentially different types of binding sites on class II molecules for alloreactive T cell receptors, direct experimental evidence for either type of ligand is lacking.

Conclusions

Our understanding of the molecular events involved in generating the trimolecular complex comprised of the T cell antigen receptor, a class II molecule and an antigen fragment have progressed significantly during the 15 years since class II molecules were identified as an important component of the ligand that initiates the antigen specific activation of T lymphocytes [9]. The tools provided by molecular biology have enabled investigators to rapidly manipulate the component molecules of this interaction and utilize what is essentially a classical genetic approach for the analysis of a biochemical problem. Selected mutants have been produced to analyze the structure-function properties of class II molecules. By analyzing these mutants, polymorphic residues have been identified that comprise antibody-binding sites, are responsible for regulating the cell surface expression of the heterodimer, control α/β chain allele-specific association and comprise alloreactive T cell receptor epitopes. The interpretation of many of these observations would be significantly enhanced if we knew the three-dimensional structure of the class II molecule. Knowledge of the crystal structure would also enable us to formulate testable hypotheses about the specific intramolecular interactions of certain class II residues.

As our understanding increases of the specific class II residues that are directly involved in T cell receptor interaction, investigators should be able to develop strategies to modulate an antigen specific immune response. By targeting on the class II antigen combining site, allele or antigen specific antagonists/agonists may be identified that can alter T cell recognition of an antigen and in vivo immune responsiveness to particular antigens.

References

1 Buus, S.; Sette, A.; Grey, H.M.: The interaction between protein-derived immunogenic peptides and Ia. Immunol. Rev. *98:* 115–141 (1987).

2 Unanue, E.R.; Allen, P.M.: The basis for the immunoregulatory role of macrophages and other accessory cells. Science *236:* 551–557 (1987).

3 Gell, P.G.H.; Benacerraf, B.: Studies on hypersensitivity. II. Delayed hypersensitivity to denatured proteins in guinea pigs. Immunology *2:* 319–343 (1959).

4 Franzl, R.E.: Immunogenic subcellular particles obtained from spleens of antigen-injected mice. Nature, Lond. *195:* 457–458 (1962).

5 Campbell, D.H.; Garvey, J.S.: Nature of retained antigen and its role in immune mechanisms. Adv. Immunol. *3:* 261–313 (1963).

6 Mosier, D.E.: A requirement for two cell types for antibody formation in vitro. Science *151:* 1573–1575 (1967).

7 Ellner, J.J.; Rosenthal, A.S.: Quantitative and immunologic aspects of the handling of 2, 4 dinitrophenyl guinea pig albumin by macrophages. J. Immun. *114:* 1563–1569 (1975).

8 Ellner, J.J.; Lipsky, P.E.; Rosenthal, A.S.: Antigen handling by guinea pig macrophages: further evidence for the sequestration of antigen relevant for activation of primed T lymphocytes. J. Immun. *118:* 2053–2057 (1977).

9 Rosenthal, A.S.; Shevach, E.M.: Function of macrophages in antigen recognition by guinea pig T lymphocytes. I. Requirement for histocompatible macrophages and lymphocytes. J. exp. Med. *138:* 1194–1212 (1973).

10 Levine, B.B.; Ojeda, A.; Benacerraf, B.: Basis for the antigenicity of hapten-poly-*L*-lysine conjugates in random bred guinea pigs. Nature, Lond. *200:* 544–546 (1963).

11 McDevitt, H.O.; Sela, M.: The genetic control of the immune response. I. Demonstration of determinant-specific differences in response to synthetic polypeptide antigens in two strains of inbred mice. J. exp. Med. *122:* 517–531 (1965).

12 McDevitt, H.O.; Benacerraf, B.: Genetic control of specific immune responses. Adv. Immunol. *11:* 31–74 (1969).

13 Rosenthal, A.S.: Determinant selection and macrophage function in genetic control of the immune response. Immunol. Rev. *40:* 136–152 (1978).

14 Ziegler, K.H.; Unanue, E.R.: Identification of a macrophage antigen processing event required for I-region-restricted antigen presentation to T lymphocytes. J. Immun. *127:* 1869–1875 (1981).

15 Shimonkevitz, R.; Kappler, J.W.; Marrack, P.; Grey, H.M.: Antigen recognition by H-2-restricted T cells. I. Cell-free antigen processing. J. exp. Med. *158:* 303–316 (1983).

16 Walden, P.; Nagy, Z.A.; Klein, J.: Induction of regulatory T-lymphocyte responses by liposomes carrying major histocompatibility complex molecules and foreign antigen. Nature, Lond. *315:* 327–329 (1985).

17 Allen, P.M.: Antigen processing at the molecular level. Immunol. Today *8:* 270–273 (1987).

18 Babbitt, B.P.; Allen, P.M.; Matsueda, G.; Haber, E.; Unanue, E.R.: Binding of immunogenic peptides to Ia histocompatibility molecules. Nature, Lond. *317:* 359–361 (1985).

19 Buus, S.; Sette, S.; Colon, S.M.; Jenis, D.M.; Grey, H.M.: Isolation and characterization of antigen-Ia complexes involved in T cell recognition. Cell *47:* 1071–1077 (1986).

20 Cresswell, P.: Intracellular class II HLA antigens are accessible to transferrin-neuraminidase conjugates internalized by receptor-mediated endocytosis. Proc. natn. Acad. Sci. USA *82:* 8188–8192 (1985).

21 Babbitt, B.P.; Matsueda, G.; Haber, E.; Unanue, E.R.; Allen, P.M.: Antigenic competition at the level of peptide-Ia binding. Proc. natn. Acad. Sci. USA *83:* 4509–4513 (1986).

22 Guillet, J.G.; Lai, M.Z.; Briner, T.J.; Buus, S.; Sette, S.; Grey, H.M.; Smith, J.A.; Gefter, M.L.: Immunological self, nonself discrimination. Science *235:* 865–870 (1987).

23 Schwartz, R.H.: Immune response (Ir) genes of the murine major histocompatibility complex. Adv. Immunol. *38:* 31–201 (1986).

24 Buus, S.; Colon, S.; Smith, C.; Freed, J.H.; Miles, C.; Grey, H.M.: Interaction between a 'processed' ovalbumin peptide and Ia molecules. Proc. natn. Acad. Sci. USA *83:* 3968–3971 (1986).

25 Bjorkman, P.J.; Saper, M.A.; Samraoui, B.; Bennett, W.S.; Strominger, J.L.; Wiley, D.C.: Structure of the human class I histocompatibility antigen, HLA-A2. Nature, Lond. *329:* 506–512 (1987).

26 Bjorkman, P.J.; Saper, M.A.; Samraoui, B.; Bennett, W.S.; Strominger, J.L.; Wiley, D.C.: The foreign antigen binding site and T cell recognition regions of class I histocompatibility antigens. Nature, Lond. *329:* 512–518 (1987).

27 Allen, P.M.; Matsueda, G.R.; Evans, R.J.; Dunbar, J.B.; Marshall, G.R.; Unanue, E.R.: Identification of the T-cell and Ia contact residues of a T-cell antigenic epitope. Nature, Lond. *327:* 713–715 (1987).

28 Rothbard, J.B.; Lechler, R.I.; Howland, K.; Bal, V.; Eckels, D.D.; Sekaly, R.; Long, E.O.; Taylor, W.R.; Lamb, J.R.: Structural model of HLA-DR1 restricted T cell antigen recognition. Cell *52:* 515–523 (1988).

29 Delisi, C.; Berzofsky, J.A.: T-cell antigenic sites tend to be amphipathic structures. Proc. natn. Acad. Sci. USA *82:* 7048–7052 (1985).

30 Heber-Katz, E.; Hollosi, M.; Dietzschold, B.; Hudeaz, F.; Fasman, G.D.: The T cell response to the glycoprotein D of the herpes simplex virus: the significance of antigen conformation. J. Immun. *135:* 1385–1390 (1985).

31 Kaufman, J.; Strominger, J.L.: HLA-DR light chain has a polymorphic n-terminal region and a conserved immunoglobulin-like C-terminal region. Nature, Lond. *297:* 694–697 (1982).

32 Jones, P.P.; Murphy, D.B.; McDevitt, H.O.: Two-gene control of the expression of murine Ia antigen. J. exp. Med. *148:* 925–939 (1978).

33 Sung, E.; Jones, P.P.: The invariant chain of murine Ia antigens: its glycosylation, abundance and subcellular localization. Mol. Immunol. *18:* 899–913 (1981).

34 McKean, D.J.; Melvold, R.W.; David, C.: Tryptic peptide comparison of Ia antigen alpha and beta polypeptides from the I-A mutant B6.C-H-2^{bm12} and its congenic parental strain B6. Immunogenetics *14:* 41–51 (1981).

35 Miller, J.; Germain, R.N.: Efficient cell surface expression of class II MHC molecules in the absence of associated invariant chain. J. exp. Med. *164:* 1478–1489 (1986).

36 Schneider, F.-J.; Opel, B.; Ballhausen, W.; Henkes, W.; Steinlein, P.; Resek, K.: Synthesis and expression of MHC class II molecules in the absence of attached invariant chains by recombinant-interferon-gamma-activated bone-marrow-derived maceophages. Eur. J. Immunol. *17:* 1235–1242 (1987).

37 Buerstedde, J.-M.; Pease, L.R.; Nilson, A.E.; Bell, M.P.; Chase, C.; Buerstedde, G.; McKean, D.J.: Regulation of murine MHC class II molecule expression: identification of A_β residues responsible for allele-specific cell surface expression. J. exp. Med. *168:* 823–837 (1988).

38 Claesson-Welsh, L.; Peterson, P.A.: Implications of the invariant gamma-chain on the intracellular transport of class II histocompatibility antigens. J. Immun. *135:* 3551–3557 (1985).

39 McNicholas, J.; Steinmetz, M.; Hunkapiller, T.; Jones, P.P.; Hood, L.: DNA sequence of the gene encoding the E alpha Ia polypeptide of the BALB/c mouse. Science *218:* 1229–1232 (1982).

40 Choi, E.; McIntyre, K.; Germain, R.N.; Seidman, J.: Murine I-A beta chain polymorphism: nucleotide sequences of three allelic I-A beta genes. Science *221:* 283–286 (1983).

41 Mengle-Gaw, L.; McDevitt, H.O.: Genetics and expression of mouse Ia antigens. A. Rev. Immunol. *3:* 367–396 (1985).

42 McKean, D.J.; Infante, A.J.; Nilson, A.; Kimoto, M.; Fathman, C.G.; Walker, E.; Warner, N.: Major histocompatibility complex-restricted antigen presentation to antigen-reactive T cells by B lymphocyte tumor cells. J. exp. Med. *154:* 1419–1413 (1981).

43 Germain, R.N.; Norcross, M.A.; Margulies, D.H.: Functional expression of a transfected murine class II MHC gene. Nature, Lond. *306:* 190–194 (1983).

44 Rabourdin-Combe, C.; Mach, B.: Expression of HLA-DR antigens at the surface of mouse L cells co-transfected with cloned human genes. Nature, Lond. *303:* 670–674 (1983).

45 Folsom, V.; Gold, D.P.; White, J.; Marrack, P.; Kappler, J.; Tonegawa, S.: Functional and inducible expression of a transfected murine class II major histocompatibility complex gene. Proc. natn. Acad. Sci. USA *81:* 2045–2049 (1984).

46 Malissen, B.; Steinmetz, M.; McMillan, M.; Pierres, M.; Hood, L.: Expression of I-A^k class II genes in mouse L cells after DNA-mediated gene transfer. Nature, Lond. *305:* 440–443 (1983).

47 Koch, N.; Harris, A.W.: Differential expression of the invariant chain in mouse tumor cells: relationship to B lymphoid development. J. Immun. *132:* 12–15 (1984).

48 Glimcher, L.H.; Polla, B.S.; Poljak, A.; Morton, C.C.; McKean, D.J.: Murine class II (Ia) molecules associate with human invariant chain. J. Immun. *138:* 1519–1523 (1987).

49 Norcross, M.A.; Bentley, D.M.; Margulies, D.H.; Germain, R.N.: Membrane Ia expression and antigen-presenting accessory cell function of L cells transfected with class II major histocompatibility complex genes. J. exp. Med. *160:* 1316–1337 (1984).

50 Malissen, B.; Price, M.P.; Goverman, J.M.; McMillan, M.; White, J.; Kappler, J.; Marrack, P.; Piettes, A.; Pierres, M.; Hood, L.: Gene transfer of H-2 class II genes: antigen presentation by mouse fibroblast and hamster B-cell lines. Cell *36:* 319–327 (1984).

51 Lechler, R.I.; Norcross, M.A.; Germain, R.N.: Qualitative and quantitative studies of antigen-presenting cell function by using I-A-expressing L cells. J. Immun. *135:* 2914–2922 (1985).

52 Cohn, L.E.; Glimcher, L.H.; Waldmann, R.A.; Smith, J.A.; Ben-Nun, A.; Seidman, J.; Choi, E.: Identification of functional regions on the I-A^b molecule by site-directed mutagenesis. Proc. natn. Acad. Sci. USA *83:* 747–751 (1986).

53 Buerstedde, J.-M.; Pease, L.R.; Bell, M.P.; Nilson, A.E.; Buerstedde, G.; Murphy, S.; McKean, D.J.: Identification of an immunodominant region on the I-A beta chain using site-directed mutagenesis and DNA-mediated gene transfer. J. exp. Med. *167:* 473–487 (1988).

54 McKenzie, I.F.C.; Morgan, G.M.; Sandrin, M.S.; Michaelides, M.M.; Melvold, R.W.; Kohn, H.I.: B6.C-H-2^{bm12}. A new H-2 mutation in the I region in the mouse. J. exp. Med. *150:* 1323–1328 (1979).

55 Hansen, T.H.; Walsh, W.D.; Ozato, K.; Arn, J.S.; Sachs, D.H.: Ia specificities on parental and hybrid cells of an I-A mutant mouse strain. J. Immun. *127:* 2228–2231 (1981).

56 Michaelidies, M.; Sandrin, M.; Morgan, G.; McKenzie, I.F.C.; Ashman, R.; Melvold, R.W.: Ir gene function in an I-A subregion mutant B6.C-H-2^{bm12}. J. exp. Med. *153:* 464–469 (1981).

57 McIntyre, K.R.; Seidman, J.: Nucleotide sequence of mutant I-A beta bm12 gene is evidence for genetic exchange between mouse immune response genes. Nature, Lond. *308:* 551–553 (1984).

58 Denaro, M.; Hammerling, U.; Rask, L.; Peterson, P.A.: The E^b gene may have acted as the donor gene in a gene conversion-like event generating the A^{bm12} beta mutant. Eur. Molec. Biol. Org. J. *3:* 2029–2032 (1984).

59 Beck, B.N.; Glimcher, L.H.; Nilson, A.E.; Pierres, M; McKean, D.J.: The structure-function relationship of I-A molecules: correlation of serologic and functional phenotypes of four I-A^k mutant cell lines. J. Immun. *133:* 3176–3182 (1984).

60 Beck, B.N.; Pease, L.R.; Bell, M.P.; Buerstedde, J.-M.; Nilson, A.E.; Schlauder, G.G.; McKean, D.J.: DNA sequence analysis of I-A^k beta mutants reveals serologically immunodominant region. J. exp. Med. *166:* 433–443 (1987).

61 Allen, P.M.; McKean, D.J.; Beck, B.N.; Sheffield, J.; Glimcher, L.H.: Direct evidence that a class II molecule and a simple globular protein generate multiple determinants. J. exp. Med. *162:* 1264–1274 (1985).

62 Beck, B.N.; Buerstedde, J.M.; Krco, C.J.; Nilson, A.E.; Chase, C.G.; McKean, D.J.: Characterization of cell lines expressing mutant I-A^b and I-A^k molecules allows the definition of distinct serologic epitopes on A alpha and A beta polypeptides. J. Immun. *136:* 2953–2961 (1986).

63 Landais, D.; Waltzinger, C.; Beck, B.N.; Staub, A.; McKean, D.J.; Benoist, C.; Mathis, D.: Functional sites on Ia molecules: a molecular dissection of A alpha immunogenicity. Cell *47:* 173–181 (1986).

64 Griffith, I.J.; Choi, E.M.; Glimcher, L.H.: A single base mutation in an I-A alpha-chain gene alters T-cell recognition. Proc. natn. Acad. Sci. USA *84:* 1090–1093 (1987).

65 Rosloniec, E.; Vitez, L.J.; Buerstedde, J.-M.; Beck, B.N.; McKean, D.J.; Landais, D.; Mathis, D.; Benoist, C.; Freed, J.: The use of antigen presenting cells bearing chimeric or mutant I-A molecules to present hen egg lysozyme fragments to T cell hybridomas reveals a functionally dominant region of the I-A^k molecule (submitted).

66 Brown, J.H.; Jardetzky, T.; Saper, M.A.; Samraoui, B.; Bjorkman, P.J.; Wiley, D.C.: A hypothetical model of the foreign antigen binding site of class II histocompatibility molecules. Nature, Lond. *332:* 845–850 (1988).

67 Griffith, I.; Carland, F.; Glimcher, L.H.: Alteration of a non-polymorphic residue in a class II E beta gene eliminates an antibody-defined epitope without affecting T cell recognition. J. Immun. *138:* 4480–4483 (1987).

68 Quill, H.; Schwartz, R.H.; Glimcher, L.H.: E^k beta mutant antigen-presenting cell lines expressing altered A^k alpha molecules. J. Immun. *136:* 3351–3359 (1986).

69 Germain, R.N.; Ashwell, J.D.; Lechler, R.I.; Margulies, D.H.; Nickerson, K.M.; Suzuki, G.; Tou, J.Y.L.: 'Exon shuffling' maps control of antibody- and T-cell-recognition sites to the NH2-terminal domain of the class II major histocompatibility polypeptide A beta. Proc. natn. Acad. Sci. USA *82:* 2940–2945 (1985).

70 Wegmann, D.R.; Roeder, W.D.; Shutter, J.R.; Kop, J.; Chiller, J.M.; Maki, R.A.: Recognition of exon-shuffled class II molecules by T helper cells. Eur. J. Immunol. *16:* 671–678 (1986).

71 Lechler, R.I.; Ronchese, F.; Braunstein, N.S.; Germain, R.N.: I-A-restricted T cell antigen recognition. Analysis of the roles of A alpha and A beta using DNA-mediated gene transfer. J. exp. Med. *163:* 678–697 (1986).

72 Braunstein, N.S.; Germain, R.N.: Allele-specific control of Ia molecule surface expression and conformation: implications for a general model of Ia structure-function relationships. Proc. natn. Acad. Sci. USA *84:* 2921–2925 (1987).

73 Beck, B.N.; Frelinger, J.G.; Shigeta, M.; Infante, A.J.; Cummings, D.; Hammerling, G.; Fathman, C.G.: T cell clones specific for hybrid I-A molecules. J. exp. Med. *156:* 1186–1194 (1982).

74 Ronchese, F.; Schwartz, R.H.; Germain, R.N.: Functionally distinct subsites on a class II major histocompatibility complex molecule. Nature, Lond. *329:* 254–256 (1987).

75 Landais, D.; Matthes, H.; Benoist, C.; Mathis, D.: A molecular basis for the Ia.2 and Ia.19 antigenic determinants. Proc. natn. Acad. Sci. USA *82:* 2930–2934 (1985).

76 Ronchese, F.; Brown, M.; Germain, R.N.: Structure-function analysis of the A^{bm12} beta mutation using site-directed mutagenesis and DNA-mediated gene transfer. J. Immun. *139:* 629–638 (1987).

77 Buerstedde, J.-M.; Nilson, A.E.; Chase, C.G.; Bell, M.P.; Beck, B.N.; Pease, L.R.; McKean, D.J.: A_β polymorphic residues responsible for class II molecule recognition by alloreactive T cells. J. exp. Med. *69:* 1645–1654 (1989).

78 Kimoto, M; Fathman, C.G.: Antigen-reactive T cell clones. I. Transcomplementing hybrid I-A-region gene products function effectively in antigen presentation. J. exp. Med. *152:* 759–770 (1980).

79 McNicholas, J.; Murphy, D.; Matis, L.A.; Schwartz, R.H.; Lerner, R.A.; Janeway, C.A., Jr.; Jones, P.P.: Immune response gene function correlates with the expression of an Ia antigen. I. Preferential association of certain Ae and E alpha chains results in a quantitative deficiency in expression of an Ae: E complex. J. exp. Med. *155:* 490–507 (1982).

80 Conrad, P.J.; Lerner, E.A.; Murphy, D.B.; Jones, P.P.; Janeway, C.A., Jr.: Differential expression of Ia glycoprotein complexes in F1 hybrid mice detected with alloreactive cloned T cell lines. J. Immun. *129:* 2616–2620 (1982).

81 Schlauder, G.G.; Bell, M.P.; Beck, B.N.; Nilson, A.; McKean, D.J.: The structure-function relationship of I-A molecules: a biochemical analysis of I-A polypeptides from mutant antigen-presenting cells and evidence of preferential association of allelic forms. J. Immun. *135:* 1945–1954 (1985).

82 Germain, R.N.; Bentley, D.M.; Quill, H.: Influence of allelic polymorphism on the assembly and surface expression of class II MHC (Ia) molecules. Cell *43:* 233–242 (1985).

83 Griffith, I.J.; Nabari, N.; Ghogawala, Z.; Chase, C.G.; Rodriguez, M.; McKean, D.J.; Glimcher, L.H.: Structural mutation affecting intracellular transport and cell surface expression of murine class II molecules. J. exp. Med. *167:* 541–555 (1988).

84 Chou, P.Y.; Fasman, G.D.: Prediction of protein conformation. Biochemistry *13:* 222–245 (1974).

85 Matzinger, P.; Bevan, M.J.: Hypothesis: why do so many lymphocytes respond to major histocompatibility antigens? Cell. Immunol. *29:* 1–5 (1977).

86 Marrack, P.; Kappler, J.: T cells can distinguish between allogeneic major histocompatibility complex products on different cell types. Nature, Lond. *332:* 840–843 (1988).
87 Glimcher, L.H.; Griffith, I.J.: Mutations of class II MHC molecules. Immunol. Today *8:* 274–279 (1987).
88 Estess, P.; Begovich, A.B.; Koo, M.; Jones, P.P.; McDevitt, H.O.: Sequence analysis and structure-function correlations of murine q, k, u, s, and f haplotype I-A beta cDNA clones. Proc. natn. Acad. Sci. USA *83:* 3590–3598 (1986).
89 Mengle-Gaw, L.; McDevitt, H.O.: Predicted protein sequence of the murine I-E-beta S-polypeptide chain from cDNA and genomic clones. Proc. natn. Acad. Sci. USA *82:* 2910–1914 (1985).

David J. McKean, PhD, Department of Immunology, Mayo Clinic,
Rochester, MN 55905 (USA)

Sercarz E (ed): Antigenic Determinants and Immune Regulation. Chem Immunol.
Basel, Karger, 1989, vol 46, pp 85–100

Insulin-Determinant Recognition by Helper and Suppressor T cells

Judith A. Kapp, Phyllis Jonas Whiteley

Department of Pathology, The Jewish Hospital of St. Louis and
Departments of Pathology and Microbiology/Immunology, Washington University
School of Medicine, St. Louis, Mo., USA

Introduction

Insulin is a protein whose amino acid sequence and tertiary structure is known. It is synthesized as a single polypeptide chain, referred to as proinsulin (fig. 1), which is cleaved by a trypsin-like enzyme in the secretory granules of the pancreatic B cells [1]. The mature insulin molecule is composed of two polypeptides, the A chain and the B chain, that are linked by disulfide bonds (fig. 1). Insulins from various mammalian species have highly conserved amino acid sequences. The substitutions that occur are generally localized to residues B3 and B30 on the B chain, the intra-chain disulfide loop region, A7-A11, and A4 of the A-chain [2]. Because most insulins are hormonally active in other species, these amino acid residues probably are not important for the hormonal activity of insulin.

Murine immune responses to heterologous insulins are controlled by MHC-linked Ir genes [3–7]. Mice bearing different H-2 haplotypes develop antibody responses to different species variants of insulin (fig. 2). Responder mice produce high levels of circulating antibodies and T cells capable of proliferating in vitro, whereas nonresponders do not. All strains of mice are able to produce insulin-specific antibodies when immunized with proinsulin [7] or insulin conjugated to the type-1, T-independent antigen, *Brucella abortus* [5]. In addition, the antibodies that are generated after immunization with one species of insulin cross-react extensively with other species of insulin, including nonimmunogenic variants [8]. Thus, the defect in nonresponder mice is not the lack of insulin-reactive B cells; rather, it is the presence or absence of functional T helper cells that determines whether a particular strain will develop antibody responses after immunization with a given insulin.

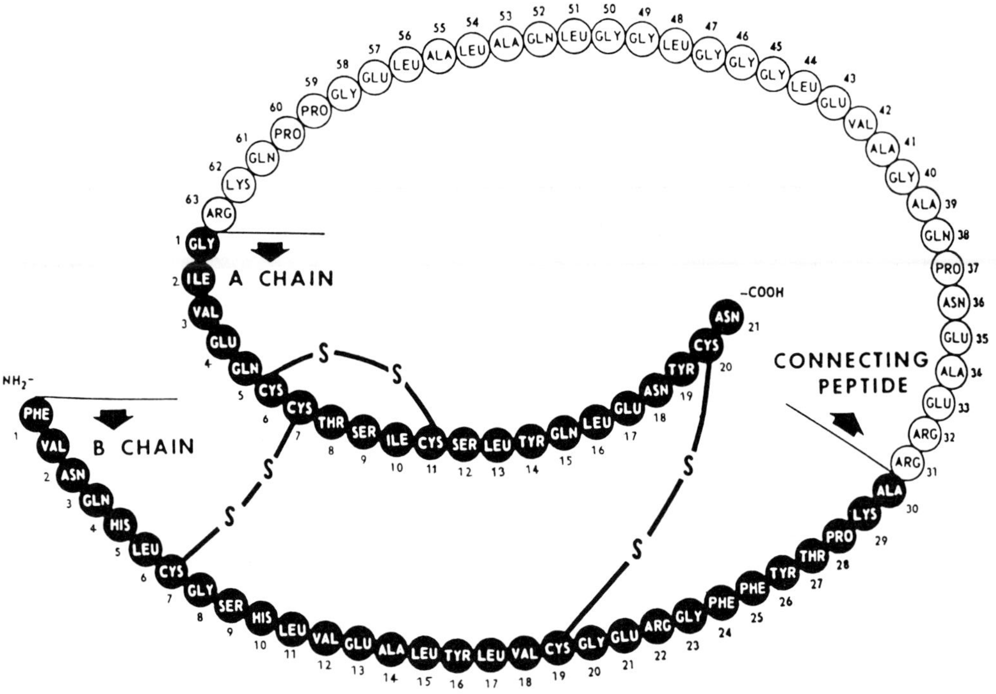

Fig. 1. Amino acid sequence of pork proinsulin. Reprinted with permission from Chance [1].

	DIFFERENCES IN AMINO ACID SEQUENCES OF INSULIN							ANTIBODY RESPONSES			
	B Chain			A Chain				by			
Species	B3	B9	B30	A4	A8	A9	A10	$H\text{-}2^d$	$H\text{-}2^b$	$H\text{-}2^k$	$H\text{-}2^q$
Mouse I	-Lys—	Pro*—	Ser-	-Asp—	Thr	Ser	Tle-	NT	NT	NT	NT
Rat I	—	—	—	—	—	—	—	–	–	–	NT
Human	-Asn—	Ser—	Thr-	-Glu—	—	—	—	+	–	–	NT
Pork	-Asn—	Ser—	Ala-	-Glu—	—	—	—	+	–	–	–
Beef	-Asn—	Ser—	Ala-	-Glu—	Ala—	—	Val-	+	+	–	–
Sheep	-Asn—	Ser—	Ala-	-Glu—	Ala	Gly	Val-	+	+	+	–
Horse	-Asn—	Ser—	Ala-	-Glu—	—	Gly—	—	+	+	+	–

Fig. 2. Amino acid sequences and immunogenicity of insulins from various species. Sequences were derived from Dayhoff [2] and responses to different species of insulin were determined by Keck [3, 4], Kapp and Strayer [7], and Bucy and Kapp [11].

Identification of the immunogenic epitopes of insulin has been more difficult than for many other proteins, primarily because T cells from mice primed with native insulin react poorly, if at all, to isolated A chains or B chains [9, 10]. Thus, it appears that the immunogenic epitope is dependent upon both chains. According to the studies of Naquet et al. [9], the minimum stimulatory fragment consists of residues A1–A14, which includes the A chain loop, linked to a B chain fragment consisting of residues B7–B15 and this fragment is processed further before presentation to Th cells. Analysis of which of these residues are involved in binding to Ia antigens and which interact with T cell receptors has not yet been reported.

Fine Specificity of Insulin-Specific Helper and Suppressor T Cells

Our studies on the mechanism of the genetic control of antibody responses to insulin raise the possibility that the pattern of responsiveness is determined by the activation and specificity of dominant Ts cells rather than by a defect in the T cell repertoire or faulty interaction of processed insulin with Ia antigens. Data supporting this interpretation will be reviewed below.

We have used a secondary adoptive transfer system [11] or a secondary Mishell-Dutton culture system [12] in which both T cells and B cells must be primed to develop insulin-specific antibody responses or hapten-specific antibody responses to haptens conjugated to insulin. C57BL/10 (B10) mice respond to beef insulin but not pork insulin in vivo [3, 6] and beef insulin-primed T cells supported responses to beef insulin, whereas pork insulin-primed T cells did not support responses to pork insulin in vitro (table 1) [12]. Because it has been shown that primed helper T (Th) cells are radioresistant, whereas unprimed helper T cells as well as primed and unprimed suppressor T (Ts) cells are radiosensitive [reviewed in ref. [13], we tested the helper activity of the insulin-primed T cells. Irradiation did not abrogate the helper activity of the T cells from beef insulin-primed mice. Irradiated, pork insulin-primed T cells provided help indicating that Th cells had been primed. The fact that unirradiated, pork insulin-primed T cells abrogated the helper activity of the irradiated T cells indicates that pork insulin primed Th cells and dominant, radiosensitive Ts cells.

Th and Ts cells can also be distinguished by the expression of cell surface antigens; Th cells are $CD4^+$ and the Ts cells are $CD8^+$ (table 2). The cross-reactivity of the primed Th cells was also examined in the experiment shown in table 2. Beef insulin-primed T cells responded to beef insulin but not to pork or mouse insulin. By contrast, the pork insulin-primed Th cells were broadly cross-reactive and responded to beef, pork,

Table 1. Pork insulin primes Th and Ts cells in B10 mice

Primed T cells[a]		Insulin	Insulin-specific PFC/culture[b]
Untreated	750R		
Beef	none	Beef	915
none	Beef	Beef	905
Beef	Beef	Beef	995
Pork	none	Pork	<10
none	Pork	Pork	600
Pork	Pork	Pork	<10

[a] Ig^- lymph node lymphocytes (2×10^6) from mice primed with the indicated insulin CFA were used as a source of T cells with or without irradiation. All cultures contained 5×10^6 splenic B cells from mice primed with Beef insulin. Cultures were stimulated with the indicated antigen.
[b] Insulin-specific PFC responses were determined on day 5.

Table 2. Fine specificity of Primed Th and Ts cells in B10 mice

Primed T cells[a]		Insulin-specific PFC/culture[b]		
$CD4^+$	$CD8^+$	Beef	Pork	mouse
Beef	none	740	10	10
none	Beef	10	10	10
Beef	Beef	810	10	10
Pork	none	680	655	655
none	Pork	10	25	nt
Pork	Pork	625	10	10

[a] Lymph node T cells (2×10^6) from mice primed with beef or pork insulin were treated with anti-Lyt 2 ($CD4^+$) or anti-Lyt 1 ($CD8^+$) antibody and complement and added to cultures containing (5×10^6) B cells from mice primed with beef insulin.
[b] Cultures were stimulated with the indicated insulin and insulin-specific PFC were determined on day 5.

and mouse insulin. The pork insulin-primed Ts cells inhibited the responses to pork and mouse insulin but not beef insulin. Pork insulin is required to activate the primed Ts cells, but even after activation they are specifically suppressive because responses to irrelevant antigens are not inhibited even in the presence of pork insulin [14]. The response of pork insulin-primed, $CD4^+$ T cells to beef insulin was not inhibited by $CD8^+$ Ts cells even in the presence of an equal concentration of pork insulin. However, this response was inhibited by Ts cells if excess pork insulin was also added to these cultures [14]. Since Ts cells are activated by low levels of pork insulin, we believe these results support the idea that Th and Ts epitopes must be covalently linked to facilitate the interaction between Th and Ts cells as elegantly demonstrated in the studies of Sercarz et al. [15]. This phenomenon is analogous to linked recognition that is required for interactions between Th cells and B cells. If antigen-specific Ts cells can take up antigen via their receptors, process it and present it to Th cells like B cells, it would explain how Ts cells which recognize native, unprocessed antigen can inhibit Th cells which recognize processed antigen in the context of self Ia. Because an excess of pork insulin is required to target pork insulin-specific Ts cells to the pork insulin-induced Th cells when they are stimulated by beef insulin, we suggest that these Th cells must have a higher avidity for beef than pork insulin.

To determine whether similar numbers of memory T cells were primed by immunogenic and nonimmunogenic insulins, various numbers of pork and beef insulin-primed $CD4^+$ T cells were mixed with a constant number of purified B cells from mice primed with fluorescein (FL) conjugated to fowl γ-globulin. Cultures were stimulated with FL-conjugated beef or pork insulin and FL-specific plaque-forming cell (PFC) responses were measured. The maximum response supported by pork insulin-primed T cells was of the same order of magnitude as that supported by beef insulin-primed T cells and titration curves of the two types of Th cells were similar (fig. 3). The same results have been obtained in vivo [16].

We also have examined the cross-reactivity patterns of Th and Ts cells in strains bearing other H-2 haplotypes [17]; the results are summarized in table 3. It is important to note that pork insulin did not activate Ts cells in strains that respond to it, such as H-2^d mice, and none of the insulin variants which stimulate antibody responses activated Ts cells in that strain. In addition to H-2^b mice, pork insulin primes Th and Ts cells in other nonresponder strains. The Th cells that are primed by pork insulin in both H-2^k and H-2^q mice react with pork insulin and cross-react with mouse insulin. Like the Th cells in H-2^b mice, those in H-2^q mice also cross-react with beef and sheep insulin; whereas those in H-2^k mice do not.

Pork insulin-primed Ts cells react with pork and mouse insulin in all strains tested. We cannot determine whether the Ts cells in H-2^k mice react with beef or sheep insulin, since pork insulin did not stimulate Th cells that react with beef or sheep insulin. The cross-reactivity pattern of pork insulin-primed Ts cells in H-2^q mice differs from the other strains, in that they are cross-reactive with all four species of insulin. Moreover, comparison of the patterns in the congenic strains, B10.A(3R) (I-A^b) and B10.A(4R) (I-A^k), with those of B10 and B10.BR mice demonstrates that (3R) responded like B10 and (4R) responded like B10.BR. Thus,

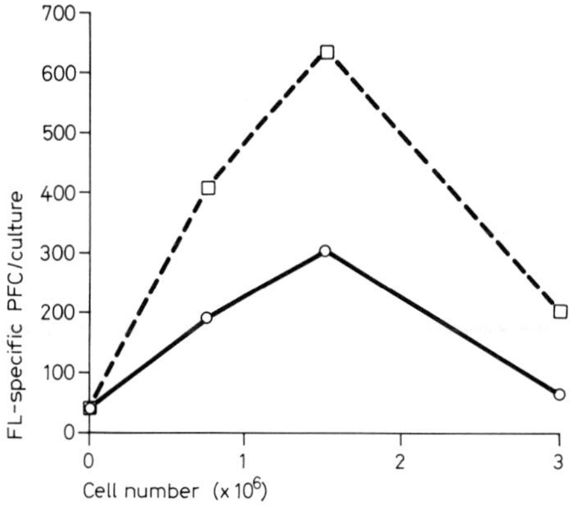

Fig. 3. In vitro titration of Th cell activity. CD4$^+$ lymph node T cells from B10 mice primed with insulin in CFA 12 days earlier were incubated with 4×10^4 FL-FGG primed syngeneic B cells. Pork insulin-primed T cells were stimulated with 1 μg/ml FL-pork insulin (○) and beef insulin-primed T cells were stimulated with 1 μg/ml FL-beef insulin (□). FL-specific PFC were enumerated 5 days later.

Table 3. Fine specificity of Th and Ts cells in mice of different H-2 haplotypes

Strain	H-2 KAED	Priming insulin	Ir	Summary of T cell activities[a]							
				helper T cells				suppressor T cells			
				beef	sheep	pork	mouse	beef	sheep	pork	mouse
BALB/c	dddd	pork	R	+	+	+	–	–	–	–	–
B10	bbbb	beef	R	+	+	–	–	–	–	–	–
B10.BR	kkkk	sheep	R	nt	+	–	–	–	–	–	–
B10	bbbb	pork	NR	+	+	+	+	–	–	+	+
B10.BR	kkkk	pork	NR	–	–	+	+	μ	μ	+	+
B10.Q	qqqq	pork	NR	+	+	+	nt	+	+	+	nt
(3R)	bbkd	pork	NR	+	+	+	+	–	–	+	+
(4R)	kkbb	pork	NR	–	–	+	+	μ	μ	+	+
b/q		pork	NR	+	+	+	nt	+	+	+	nt

[a] The helper and suppressor activity of T cells from the indicated responder (R) and nonresponder (NR) strains of mice were assayed according to the protocol described in table 1 or table 2. The results are summarized by the following symbols: (+) detectable activity; (–) no detectable activity; (μ) activity could not be determined; (nt) not tested.

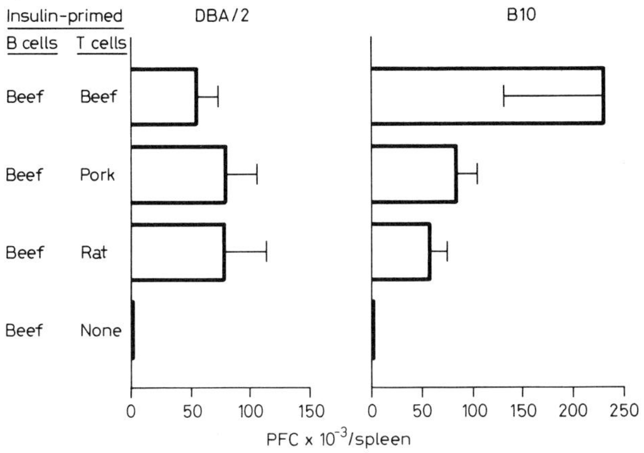

Fig. 4. Priming of Th cells by various species of insulin. Lymph node T cells (10^7) from DBA/2 (H-2d) or B10 (H-2b) mice primed with 50 μg of beef, pork, or rat insulin in CFA were transferred with 20×10^6 syngeneic beef insulin-primed splenic B cells into syngeneic recipients that had been irradiated with 650 rad. One day later mice were injected i.p. with 50 μg beef insulin in CFA, and 9 days later insulin-specific splenic PFC were enumerated.

the cross-reactivity pattern of Th and Ts cells is controlled by the I-A subregion of the MHC. The pattern seen in (B10 × B10.Q)F1 hybrids is the same as that of the B10.Q parent suggesting that broad cross-reactivity is dominant. The F1 hybrid combination between H-2^b and H-2^k is uninformative as this F1 responds to pork insulin because of complementation between the α and β chains of the I-A antigens [16, 17]. The observations that: (1) heterologous insulins that cross-react with mouse insulin are nonimmunogenic, and (2) cross-reactivity patterns of Th and Ts cells are controlled by MHC-linked genes support the idea that major histocompatibility complex (MHC)-linked nonresponsiveness is mechanistically related to self-tolerance [18]. However, our data suggest that Th cells which recognize certain autologous antigens are not physically eliminated from the system, rather they are functionally attenuated by dominant, Ts cells that are also specific for the autologous antigen.

The regulatory T cells that are stimulated by heterologous, pork insulin are not cross-reactive with mouse insulin but can be directly activated by injection of autologous insulin as shown using an adoptive transfer model [6]. In this experiment, lymph node T cells from mice primed with beef, pork or rat insulin were transferred with beef insulin-primed B cells into irradiated, syngeneic mice. In this experiment, the T cells were not irradiated or treated with antibody to deplete the Ts cells; thus, cross-reactive help was measured by challenging all of the recipient

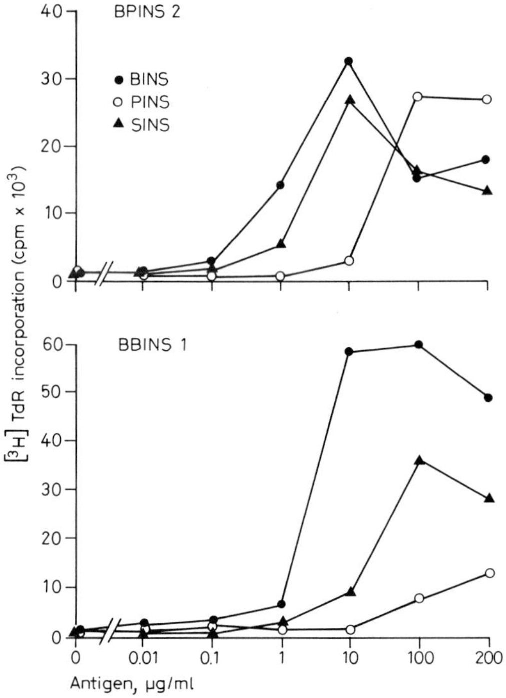

Fig. 5. Dose-response curves of BPINS 2 (upper) and BBINS 1 (lower) to various species of insulin. T cells at 2×10^4 cells per well ere cultured for 4 days with 10^6 irradiated syngeneic splenic antigen-presenting cells and various doses of beef (●), pork (○), or sheep (▲) insulin. Four hours prior to harvesting, [3H]thymidine was added to each well.

mice with beef insulin. Insulin-specific, splenic PFC were measured (fig. 4). We used rat insulin, which is identical in amino acid sequence to mouse insulin, rather than mouse insulin to prime T cells in this experiment because we did not have sufficient mouse insulin. The data clearly show that rat insulin-primed Th cells cross-react with beef insulin in both $H\text{-}2^b$ and $H\text{-}2^d$ mice. Irradiated, rat insulin-primed T cells from B10 mice also have been shown to provide Th activity when stimulated with beef, pork or mouse insulin in vitro [19].

Comparison of Insulin-Specific T Cell Lines and Clones

Based on the fact that memory Th cells were detected with approximately equal frequency among T cells from B10 mice primed with beef or pork insulin, we established long-term antigen-specific T cell lines from

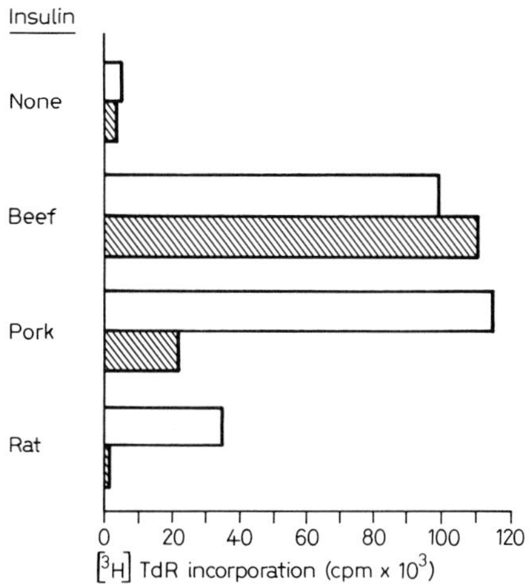

Fig. 6. Proliferative responses to rat insulin. BPINS 2 (■) and BBINS (▨) were stimulated with 100 μg/ml of the indicated insulin as described in figure 5. Reprinted with permission from Whiteley et al. [16].

these primed lymph node T cells using traditional techniques [15]. Dose-dependent proliferative responses of the resulting lines were determined (fig. 5) [16]. The pork insulin-induced line, BPINS 2, responded to beef, sheep, and pork insulin. This line is heteroclitic as it responds to beef and sheep insulin at lower doses than the immunizing antigen, pork insulin. This observation supports our idea that pork insulin-primed Th cells express higher avidity for beef than pork insulin. Clones derived from BPINS 2 also cross-react with beef, sheep, and pork insulin (not shown). The line derived from beef insulin-primed B10 mice, BBINS 1, responded to beef and sheep insulin. Shortly after this line was established, a low but reproducible proliferative response could be stimulated by very high doses of pork insulin; however, this low response was completely lost from this line during a few months of continuous culture. Clones derived from BBINS 1 also respond to beef and sheep but not pork insulin. The maximum proliferative responses by BBINS 1 and BPINS 2 were stimulated by same dose of beef insulin (10 μg/ml) which suggests that there is no difference in the avidity between the pork and beef insulin-primed Th cells.

We also tested the proliferative responses of the two lines to rat insulin; BPINS 2 responded but BBINS 1 did not (fig. 6). The dose of insulin in this experiment was 100 μg/ml, which is in excess of the dose

Table 4. Pork insulin primed clone provides help and is susceptible to suppressor T cells

Pork insulin-primed[a]		Insulin	FL-specific PFC/culture[b]
BPINS2	Ts cells		
+	–	none	245
+	–	FL-pork	2,840 (100)
+	+	FL-pork	515 (18)
+	–	FL-beef	2,765 (100)
+	+	FL-beef	2,420 (88)

[a] All cultures contained 5×10^6 FL-ovalbumin primed B10 B cells and 2×10^4 BPINS 2 cells. $CD8^+$ T cells (2×10^6 cells/culture) from pork insulin-primed B10 mice were used as a source of Ts cells. Cultures were stimulated with the indicated antigens.
[b] FL-specific PFC were determined; numbers in parentheses are percent of control.

required to stimulate maximum responses to beef and/or pork insulin. Higher doses of rat insulin have not be tested nor have responses to rat insulin by T cell clones been tested because of the limited availability of the antigen. The proliferative responses by BPINS 2 and BBINS 1, as well as the clones derived from them, are MHC-restricted and map to the I-A subregion (not shown).

The insulin-specific T cell lines and clones derived from them behave like classical Th cells in that they secrete lymphokines after activation with antigen and the appropriate antigen-presenting cells which support the growth of the cell line, CTLL (not shown). These T cell lines also provide cognate help to B cells for development of PFC responses in vitro [16]. A representative experiment in which B cells from FL-primed B10 mice were cultured with BPINS 2 and stimulated with FL-insulin is shown in table 4. BPINS 2 supported responses to both FL-pork and FL-beef insulin as expected from the proliferative responses to this cell line. Addition of pork insulin-primed lymph node T cells to these cultures inhibited the response to FL-pork insulin but not FL-beef insulin. The response to FL-beef insulin could be inhibited if excess pork insulin was also included in the culture (not shown).

Conclusions

The data described above show that insulin-specific Th cells can be demonstrated in pork insulin-primed nonresponder mice if primed Ts cells are deleted. Moreover, Th cells can be readily cloned from pork insulin-primed nonresponder mice and such clones are functionally indistinguishable from those induced by beef insulin. Both are MHC-restricted, $CD4^+$ cells that proliferate, produce lymphokines and provide carrier-specific help to B cells. These observations refute the possibility that the Th cell activity, which is normally masked by Ts cells in nonresponder mice, constitutes the activity of a different type of Th cell that those stimulated by an immunogenic variant of insulin. In addition, the frequency of memory Th cells primed by pork insulin is approximately equal to that primed by beef insulin arguing against the likelihood that clones derived from pork insulin-primed mice might represent a rare cell that was fortuitously selected and expanded during the culturing procedure. Thus, we have been unable to discern any qualitative or quantitative differences in helper activity of T cells primed with pork or beef insulin. Abromson-Leeman et al. [20] also have cloned insulin-specific Th cells from nonresponder mice; these clones were derived from B10.A mice primed with beef insulin but were said not to respond to rat insulin.

If the Th cells primed with nonimmunogenic variants of insulin are not quantitatively or qualitatively different than those stimulated by immunogenic variants, we must ask how suppression becomes dominant in nonresponder mice? This is a particularly important issue because Ts cells can be stimulated by virtually any immunogen provided it is administered under the appropriate conditions, such as in low doses or in the absence of adjuvant [21]. Once the Ts cells have been activated and/or expanded they can interfere with the activity of virgin and memory Th cells. It seems as if there is a critical balance between Th and Ts cells and once the balance is altered in one direction or the other by antigen, it remains stable at the new level. Thus, we could envision that Ts cells express antigen-specific receptors that arising by random rearrangement of gene segments, like immunoglobulins or TcR, and that those Ts cells bearing receptors for autologous proteins normally encountered during circulation in the periphery become activated and expanded. Therefore, Ts cells specific for autologous antigens would be dominant prior to exposure to exogenous antigen. Any heterologous antigen that cross-reacted with Ts cells specific for an autologous antigen would be perceived as nonimmunogenic even when administered with adjuvant because the balance of Th and Ts cells would already favor Ts cells. However, it is important to remember that these Ts cells must be activated by antigen to cause suppression and that activated Ts cells do not inhibit the priming of Th cells, but only interfere with their function. This model predicts that if the balance of Ts and Th cells specific for an autologous antigen should be reversed by some process such as a viral infection, an autoimmune response could develop should the Th cells become activated.

Our data demonstrate that Th cells induced by nonimmunogenic variants of insulin recognize antigen complexed with autologous Ia antigens. These observations provide evidence against strict clonal deletion and determinant selection models to explain H-2-linked unresponsiveness in this system. However, close examination of the cross-reactivity patterns of Th cells indicates that immunogenic and nonimmunogenic variants of insulin do not activate the same Th cell clones. All of the clones from B10 mice primed with the immunogenic beef insulin recognized beef but not pork insulin. The epitope recognized by these T cells most likely involves the disulfide-bonded loop region of the A chain, since this is the only difference in amino acid sequence between beef and pork insulin. The fact that the bulk cell line from beef insulin-primed B10 mice originally contained some cells cross-reactive with pork, but not mouse insulin suggests that some rare clones may recognize one of the three amino acids that are shared by beef and pork insulin but differ from mouse insulin. On the other hand, the pork insulin-primed lines and clones derived from nonresponder B10 mice are cross-reactive for beef, pork, sheep, and rat insulin. A critical, as yet unanswered question, raised by these studies is why injection of beef insulin does not also prime the clones which recognize the cross-reactive determinant, since the clones primed by pork insulin clearly respond to beef insulin? The answer is currently unknown; however, the possibility that beef insulin primes Ts cells capable of inhibiting responses by the cross-reacting T cells has been eliminated [14]. Although the antigenic epitope that is recognized by the cross-reactive clones remains to be determined, it might be one of numerous determinants that are shared between the heterologous and autologous insulins. Alternatively, these Th cells might recognize a determinant involving the loop region of the A chain, like Th cells stimulated by immunogenic variants [11], but the cross-reactive Th cells would be unable to discriminate between the different sequences in the loop region of beef, pork, sheep or mouse insulin.

The observation that an antigen under Ir gene control stimulates Th and Ts cells which recognize an autologous antigen in nonresponder strains supports the hypothesis that MHC-linked nonresponsiveness to certain antigens involves the mechanisms that maintain self-tolerance. Our data also show that Th cells which recognize autologous proteins may not be clonally deleted from the system if they can be functionally attenuated by autoreactive Ts cells. The overall significance of our observations will depend upon how representative they are. Experiments are currently in progress to determine whether other nonimmunogenic forms of insulin such as beef insulin primes Th and Ts cells that cross-react with autologous insulin in nonresponder mice.

Additional data which support our model can be derived from studies on autoimmunity. For example, T cells from approximately 20% of diabetics treated with heterologous insulin develop strong proliferative responses when stimulated by beef or pork insulin and a significant percentage of these also respond to human insulin [22]. In addition, T cells that react with autoantigens, such as the acetylcholine receptor [23] and autologous thymocytes [24] have been cloned from patients with spontaneous autoimmune diseases. T cells specific for autologous antigens such as collagen [25], myelin basic protein [26], and thyroglobulin [27] also have been cloned from animals in which autoimmune disease when transferred to normal, syngeneic recipients [25–27]. Since there is no evidence that the antigenic specificity of T cell receptors can be altered by somatic mutation [28], the T cells which recognize autologous proteins must have escaped clonal deletion.

The data of Kappler et al. [29, 30] demonstrate that T cells bearing receptors for MHC class II (I-E) antigen and the minor lymphocyte stimulating antigen, Mls, are detectable among the immature cells in the thymus but not in the periphery of mice expressing the relevant I-E or Mls antigen. These observations suggest that the relevant clones were deleted in the thymus. If clonal deletion is the primary mechanism for maintaining tolerance to all self antigens, then the T cells that recognize autologous antigens in our system and in autoimmune diseases would have to be the progeny of T cells which escaped clonal deletion in the thymus. One explanation for T cells escaping clonal deletion might be that they are rare cells which express receptors of low avidity. Arguing against this interpretation is our data showing that: (1) immunogenic and nonimmunogenic insulins prime similar numbers of memory T cells, and (2) the dose of antigen required to stimulate proliferation of clones derived from these memory T cells is of the same order of magnitude for immunogenic and nonimmunogenic insulins. These data suggest that T cells with receptors specific for certain autologous antigens are not deleted in the thymus.

In our opinion, there is a simple explanation for the seemingly conflicting data on clonal deletion of T cells which recognize autologous antigens. Clonal deletion is an antigen-dependent event; thus, autologous proteins must reach the thymus in sufficient quantities to cause deletion of the relevant clones. It is clear that T cells specific for autologous antigens which are synthesized in the thymus itself, such as MHC class II antigens, are deleted in the thymus. Similarly, it can be expected that T cells specific for other self-proteins will also be deleted if these proteins reach the thymus. We propose that T cells specific for self-proteins that are not encountered in the thymus, as well as those recognizing exogenous proteins, would not be deleted. Moreover, the Th cells specific for autologous antigens that emigrate to the periphery may be directly involved in expansion of the Ts cell subset specific for the same autologous protein. This model is consistent with all of the data and, furthermore, it is a testable model.

To directly address the issue of how self-tolerance to insulin is generated, we have used mice that are transgenic for the human insulin gene. These mice express mRNA encoding human insulin only in the β cells of the pancreas and they synthesize both mouse and human insulin in response to normal physiological signals [31]. Because the strain of mice used as recipients of the human insulin gene normally respond to human insulin, the transgenic mice clearly have Ia antigens that can properly associate with human insulin and the genetic capacity to produce Th cells with receptors which recognize human insulin. The data indicate that the transgenic mice are tolerant to human insulin, whereas syngeneic, nontransgenic littermates mount a normal immune response to human insulin [Whiteley et al., submitted]. Nevertheless, human insulin primes Th cells specific for human insulin that can be hybridized to BW5147 with equal efficiency in transgenic and nontransgenic littermates. This observation suggests that acquired tolerance to human insulin is not the result of clonal deletion and raises the possibility that it may be maintained by the development of Ts cells specific for human insulin. This interpretation is currently under investigation. To date, the information from the transgenic mice is entirely comparable to the observations derived from nonresponder mice injected with pork insulin and thus provides strong support for our explanation for the appearance of mature Th cells which recognize certain autologous proteins in peripheral lymphoid organs.

Acknowledgements

This work was supported in part by US Public Health Service Basic Science Research Grant and Grant AI-13987 from the National Institute of Allergy and Infectious Diseases, US Public Health Service Training Grant AI-07163, and US Public Health Service Diabetes Research and Training Center Grant 2P60 DK20579.

References

1 Chance, R.E.: Amino acid sequences of proinsulins and intermediates. Diabetes *21:* suppl. 2, pp. 461–467 (1972).
2 Dayhoff, M.O.: Atlas of protein sequences and structure. *5:* D208 (1972).
3 Keck, K.: Ir gene control of immunogenicity of insulin and A-chain loop as a carrier determinant. Nature, Lond. *254:* 78–79 (1975).

4 Keck, K.: Ir gene control of carrier recognition. III. Cooperative recognition of two or more carrier determinants on insulins of different species. Eur. J. Immunol. *7:* 811–816 (1977).
5 Thomas, J.W.; Bucy, R.P.; Kapp, J.A.: T cell-independent responses to an Ir gene-controlled antigen. I. Characteristics of the immune response to *Brucella abortus*. J. Immun. *129:* 6–10 (1982).
6 Kapp, J.A.; Bucy, R.P.: Ir gene control of the insulin-specific immune response in mice; in Keck, Erb, Basic and clinical aspects of immunity to insulin, pp. 71–80 (de Gruyter, Berlin 1981).
7 Kapp, J.A.; Strayer, D.S.: H-2 linked Ir gene control of antibody responses to porcine insulin. I. Development of insulin-specific antibodies in some but not all nonresponder strains injected with proinsulin. J. Immun. *121:* 978–982 (1978).
8 Kapp, J.A.; Strayer, D.S.; Robbins, P.F.; Perlmutter, R.M.: Insulin-specific murine antibodies of limited heterogeneity. I. Genetic control of spectrotypes. J. Immun. *123:* 109–114 (1979).
9 Naquet, P.; Ellis, J.; Baghirath, S.; Hodges, R.S.; Delovitch, T.L.: Processing and presentation of insulin. I. Analysis of immunogenic peptides and processing requirements for insulin A chain loop specific T cells. J. Immun. *139:* 3955–3963 (1988).
10 Glimcher, L.H.; Schroer, J.A.; Chan, C.; Shevach, E.M.: Fine specificity of cloned insulin-specific T cell hybridomas: evidence supporting a role for tertiary conformation. J. Immun. *131:* 2868–2874 (1983).
11 Bucy, R.P.; Kapp, J.A.: Ir gene control of the immune response to insulins. I. Pork insulin stimulates T cell activity in nonresponder mice. J. Immun. *126:* 603–607 (1981).
12 Jensen, P.E.; Kapp, J.A.: Regulatory mechanisms of the immune response to heterologous insulins. I. Development and regulation of plaque-forming cells in vitro. Cell. Immunol. *87:* 73–84 (1984).
13 Katz, D.H.: Lymphocyte differentiation and regulation, pp. 315–345 (Academic Press, New York 1977).
14 Jensen, P.E.; Pierce, C.W.; Kapp, J.A.: Regulatory mechanisms in immune responses to heterologous insulins. II. Suppressor T cell activation associated with nonresponsiveness in H-2^b mice. J. exp. Med. *160:* 1012–1026 (1984).
15 Sercarz, E.E.; Yowell, R.L.; Turkin, D.; Miller, A.; Araneo, B.A.; Adorini, L.: Different functional specificity repertoires for suppressor and helper T cells. Immunol. Rev. *39:* 108 (1978).
16 Whiteley, P.J.; Jensen, P.E.; Pierce, C.W.; Abruzzini, A.F.; Kapp, J.A.: Helper T-cell clones that recognize autologous insulin are stimulated in nonresponder mice by pork insulin. Proc. natn. Acad. Sci. USA *85:* 2723–2727 (1988).
17 Jensen, P.E.; Kapp, J.A.: Genetics of insulin-specific helper and suppressor T cells in nonresponder mice. J. Immun. *135:* 2990–2995 (1985).
18 Schwartz, R.H.: A clonal deletion model for Ir gene control of the immune response. Scand. J. Immunol. *7:* 3–10 (1978).
19 Jensen, P.E.; Kapp, J.A.: Stimulation of helper T cells and dominant suppressor T cells that recognize autologous insulin. J. mol. cell. Immunol. *2:* 133–139 (1985).
20 Abromson-Leeman, S.; Laning, J.; Cantor, H.; Dorf, M.E.: Isolation of antigen-specific T cell clones from nonresponder mice. Eur. J. Immunol. *18:* 145–152 (1988).
21 Dorf, M.E.; Benacerraf, B.: Suppressor cells and immunoregulation. A. Rev. Immunol. *2:* 127–157 (1984).
22 Nell, L.J.; Virta, V.J.; Thomas, J.W.: Recognition of human insulin in vitro by T cells from subjects treated with animal insulins. J. clin. Invest. *76:* 2070–2077 (1988).
23 Hohlfield, R.; Toyka, K.V.; Meininger, K.; Grosse-Wilde, H.; Kalies, I.: Autoimmune

human T lymphocytes specific for acetylcholine receptor. Nature, Lond. *310:* 244–246 (1985).
24 MacKenzie, W.A.; Schwartz, A.E.; Friedman, E.W.; Davies, T.F.: Intrathyroidal T cell clones from patients with autoimmune thyroid disease J. clin. Endocr. Metab. *64:* 818–824 (1987).
25 Holmdahl, R.; Klareskog, L.; Rubin, K.; Larsson, E.; Wigzell, H.: T lymphocytes in collagen II-induced arthritis in mice. Scand. J. Immunol. *22:* 295–306 (1985).
26 Zamvil, S.S.; Mitchell, D.J.; Moore, A.C.; Kitamura, K.; Steinman, L.; Rothbard, J.B.: T-cell epitope of the autoantigen myelin basic protein that includes encephalomyelitis. Nature, Lond. *324:* 258–260 (1986).
27 Romball, C.G.; Weigle, W.O.: Transfer of experimental autoimmune thyroiditis with T cell clones. J. Immun. *138:* 1092–1098 (1987).
28 Kronenberg, M.; Siu, G.; Hood, L.E.; Shastri, N.: The molecular genetics of the T-cell antigen receptor and T-cell antigen recognition. A. Rev. Immunol. *4:* 529–592 (1986).
29 Kappler, J.W.; Roehm, N.; Marrack, P.: Tolerance by clonal elimination in the thymus. Cell *49:* 273–280 (1987).
30 Kappler, J.W.; Staerz, U.; White, J.; Marrack, P.: Self-tolerance eliminates T cells specific for Mls-modified products of the major histocompatibility complex. Nature, Lond. *332:* 35–40 (1988).
31 Selden, R.F.; Skoskiewicz, M.J.; Howie, K.B.; Russell, P.S.; Goodman, H.M.: Nature, Lond. *321:* 525–528 (1986).

Judith A. Kapp, PhD, Department of Pathology, The Jewish Hospital of St. Louis and Departments of Pathology and Microbiology/Immunology, Washington University School of Medicine, St. Louis, MO 63110 (USA)

Sercarz E (ed): Antigenic Determinants and Immune Regulation. Chem Immunol.
Basel, Karger, 1989, vol 46, pp 101–125

Encephalitogenic Epitopes of Myelin Basic Protein

Robert B. Fritz, Dale E. McFarlin[1]

Department of Microbiology and Immunology, Emory University, Atlanta, Ga.; Neuroimmunology Branch, National Institute of Neurological and Communicative Disorders and Stroke, National Institutes of Health, Bethesda, Md., USA

Encephalitogenic Antigens

Within 3 years after the introduction of attenuated rabies vaccine by Pasteur in 1885 reports of neurological sequelae related to this treatment began to appear [Gonzalez, 1888]. By 1905, a sufficient number of cases of postvaccinal encephalomyelitis had occurred to warrant a review of this procedure. Considerable controversy existed concerning the relationship of neurological complications and the attenuated rabies virus used for vaccination [Remlinger, 1905]. In order to circumvent the issue of live virus, Semple introduced a killed virus vaccine in 1919. Although the killed vaccine prevented rabies, neurological complications persisted [Stuart, 1928; Witebsky, 1928]. Recipients of the vaccine developed antibodies which reacted with brain extracts which suggested that the neurological complications were due to sensitization by nervous system antigens associated with the virus preparation.

The pioneer experiments of Rivers et al. [1933] established this point experimentally. Repeated injections of CNS extracts into monkeys reproduced postvaccinal encephalomyelitis. Neuropathological examination of affected animals showed extensive areas of myelin destruction associated with perivenular infiltration of lymphocytes and monocytes.

Initially, induction of the experimental correlate of postvaccinal encephalomyelitis, experimental allergic encephalomyelitis (EAE), required multiple injections of CNS extracts, but Morgan [1947] and Kabat [1947] were able to produce the disease by a single injection of CNS extract in adjuvant. Chemical characterization of the encephalitogen [Laatsch et al., 1962] showed that the antigen resided in myelin, and it was subsequently

[1] The authors thank Dr. Russell Martenson for his assistance with MBP sequences.

demonstrated that purified myelin basic protein (MBP) was capable of induction of the disease [Kies, 1965].

Other components of myelin, including proteolipid protein and lipids are antigenic and following immunization with whole CNS preparations, immune reactivity to multiple antigens likely contributes to the disorder. Indeed, it has been demonstrated that purified proteolipid protein is encephalitogenic in rats and mice [Yamamura et al., 1986; Trotter et al., 1987; Satoh et al., 1987]. Very recently, an encephalitogenic region of this antigen has been identified [Tuohy et al., 1988].

Pathogenesis of EAE

Existing data indicate that EAE is mediated by antigen-specific T cells [Waksman and Morrison, 1951]. The initial report by Paterson [Paterson, 1960] that adoptive transfer of EAE was mediated by immune cells, but not antibody, has been followed by numerous reports which have confirmed this finding [Stone, 1961; Panitch and McFarlin, 1977; Driscoll et al., 1979; Richert et al., 1979, 1985; Ben-Nun et al., 1981a, b; Ben-Nun and Lando, 1983; Vandenbark et al., 1985]. Further, in rats and mice the $L3T4^{+}$ subset of T cells is responsible for disease induction [Pettinelli and McFarlin, 1981; Holda and Swanborg, 1982; Lemire et al., 1986], and T cell clones that adoptively transfer disease in SJL/J and PL/J mice have been described [Zamvil et al., 1985a, b; Sakai et al., 1986]. Collectively, these data indicate that the minimal requirement for disease is a sensitized clone of T cells. However, it is likely in fully developed EAE, particularly the chronic, relapsing models induced with whole CNS tissue, that other types of immune reactivity contribute. From the point of view of the T cell the pathogenetic process can be considered in three stages: (1) the initial event leading to sensitization of T cells; (2) the migration of sensitized T cells to the CNS, and (3) reaction of the sensitized T cells with the target tissue with resultant damage.

Variables in the Production of EAE

EAE has been produced in many mammalian species by a variety of techniques. This has resulted in a number of different models which vary clinically, pathologically, and probably in terms of pathogenesis. Several variables are critical in the disease process. It cannot be emphasized too strongly that the interplay of multiple known (and unknown) variables strongly influences the immune response to encephalitogens and expression

Table 1. Variables in the induction of allergic experimental encephalomyelitis

Animals
Species
Genetics
Age
Presence of endogenous infectious agents (e.g. mouse hepatitis virus, Sendai virus)
Immunogen
Whole CNS tissue
Myelin
Myelin basic protein
MBP peptides
Site and number of injections
Adjuvants
Species of Mycobacteria used
B. pertussis source
Stress
Environmental conditions in animal rooms

of clinical EAE. Failure to recognize this has led to confusing results and conflicting claims in the literature. Many of the conflicts can be resolved if the experimental conditions used in different laboratories are carefully examined.

It is important to emphasize at this point that EAE is not the result of some mystical phenomenon, but rather follows the rules of immunology as we know them. Sometimes this is not clear particularly in early studies of EAE performed before modern immunological concepts evolved. The immune response to MBP, the initiating step of the encephalitogenic process is under immune response (IR) gene control [Fritz et al., 1983c; 1985a]. As with all responses under this type of control a spectrum of variables influences the result. Some of the important variables are discussed below and summarized in table 1.

Host Factors

Of prime importance is the animal species being studied. The genetic constitution of the host is important, with the degree of inbreeding and the age of the animal critical variables. In outbred animals susceptibility and manifestations of the disease vary considerably. In spite of this a considerable amount of research has been conducted in outbred rabbits, guinea

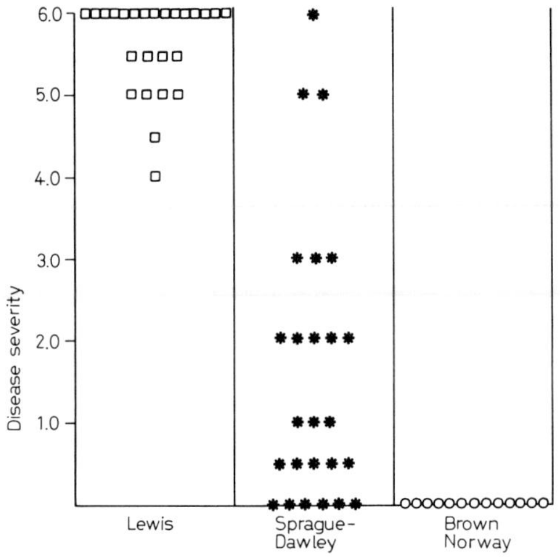

Fig. 1. Experimental allergic encephalomyelitis in Lewis ($RT1^l$), Sprague-Dawley ($RT1^w$) and Brown Norway ($RT1^n$) rats following immunization with 50 μg of myelin basic protein in complete adjuvant.

pigs, rats and primates. The latter are of particular value in attempting to understand changes that might be relevant to human disease such as shifts in blood lymphocyte phenotypes and for evaluation of experimental therapeutic modalities.

Certain inbred strains of rats, guinea pigs and mice are susceptible while others are relatively resistant. For example, outbred Sprague-Dawley rats vary in the expression of clinical disease, while inbred Lewis rats are uniformly susceptible and manifest maximal clinical disease. In contrast, Brown Norway rats are relatively resistant and do not develop disease when immunized under the same conditions (fig. 1) [Gasser et al., 1973; Williams and Moore, 1973]. Inbred strain 13 guinea pigs are susceptible to EAE whereas strain 2 animals are relatively resistant [Stone, 1961; Webb et al., 1973a, b; Teitelbaum et al., 1977; Ben-Nun et al., 1981a, b]. The term relatively resistant is used since EAE may be induced in 'resistant' strains by modification of the immunization procedure [Levine and Sowinski, 1975].

Over the past decade the mouse has become one of the major investigative models for EAE; however, a problem with this species has been the inconsistent response of 'susceptible' strains. Frequently, only a fraction of the immunized mice showed signs of clinical disease. This has led to the use of different inocula and additional adjuvants to maximize disease expression.

Table 2. Susceptibility of inbred strains of mice to MBP-induced EAE[a]

Strain	Ia	EAE	Epitope[b]
PL/J	u	+	a
A/J	k	++	a
SJL/J	s	++	b
SWR/J	q	+	b
DBA1/J	q	+	b
A.SW/J	s	+	b
B10.A	k	+	a
B10.PL(73NS)	u	+++	a
B10.T(6R)	q	++	b
B10	b	—	—
BALB/C	d	—	—
(SJL × PL)F1	s/u	+++	a

[a] When animals are immunized with MBP or MBP peptide emulsified in Freund's incomplete adjuvant supplemented with 1 mg/ml *M. tuberculosis* H37Ra and injected with 1×10^{10} killed *B. pertussis* organisms 24 and 72 h after immunization.
[b] Epitope a is in N-terminal region; epitope b is in C-terminal region of MBP molecule. Only the epitopes for PL, SJL and (SJL × PL)F1 have been precisely determined.

A number of mouse strains have been surveyed for the capacity to develop EAE [Levine and Sowinski, 1973, 1975; Yasuda et al., 1975; Bernard, 1976; Lando et al., 1979; Raine et al., 1980; Linthicum and Frelinger, 1982; Montogomery and Rauch, 1982]. Although the methods varied in different studies, the inoculum consisted of spinal cord homogenate (SCH) because under the conditions employed MBP was less potent. Since the use of such a heterogeneous inoculum makes interpretation of the genetics of the immune response difficult, this question was approached by immunization with MBP or peptides derived from the protein [Fritz et al., 1983c, 1985a]. Table 2 shows the susceptibility and epitope specificity of a few representative strains of mice following immunization with MBP or MBP peptides.

Over 40 inbred, MHC-congenic, and mutant strains of mice have been tested for susceptibility to MBP-induced EAE [Fritz, unpublished]. The majority were found to be resistant or weakly susceptible. The most susceptible strain under our conditions of immunization was the B10.PL(73NS). Routinely 90% or greater of the immunized animals developed signs of clinical EAE within 14–21 days after injection. These data are summarized in table 3.

Table 3. Susceptibility[a] of various inbred, MHC-congenic and mutant mouse strains to experimental allergic encephalomyelitis

Very susceptible	Susceptible	Resistant
Inbred		
B10.PL(73NS) B10.RIII	A/J, A/Wy/Sn, C57L, PL/J, SJL/J, DBA1/J, SWR/J, C3H/HeJ, B10.A B10.D2, A.SW, B10.A(4R), B10.T(6R), B10.MBR	BALB/c, C57BL/6 C57BL/10, MRL B10.M, B10.BR, A.BY, A.TH, A.TL B10.SM, B10.S, B10.A(5R), bml bm3, bm12, dml dm2
F1 Hybrid		
PL × SJL, SJL × PL, B10.PL × B10.S,	SJL × DBA/1, PL × DBA/1 SJL × B6, SJL × B10, PL × SWR, B10.PL × B10	BALB/c × SJL, B10 × B10.A

[a] Animals were immunized as described in table 1.

Immunogen

A second variable is the encephalitogenic inoculum. In some instances whole CNS tissue composed of a large number of antigens was administered, and in others purified components such as MBP or a fragment of MBP prepared either by proteolytic cleavage or peptide synthesis were used. The expression and intensity of disease can be related to this variable This is particularly true in the case of outbred guinea pigs. Homogenate of whole CNS tissue produces a more reproducible and severe disease as assessed by both clinical and pathological criteria. Immunizaton with a synthetic encephalitogenic peptide induces disease even milder than that obtained with MBP.

Significant differences also exist in the response of mice to whole CNS tissue or purified MBP. For example, certain strains of mice are resistant to MBP-induced EAE but not CNS tissue-induced EAE. The opposite also occurs. In fact, A.SW and B10.T(6R) mice are resistant to MBP-induced EAE, but immunization with the C-terminal half of the MBP will induce clinical disease [Fritz et al., 1985a]. Resistance and susceptibility, then, are relative terms dependent upon the antigen used as well as the strain and species being studied.

The source of the CNS tissue or MBP preparation is important in some species. For example, in highly susceptible Lewis rats bovine CNS preparations and bovine MBP are less encephalitogenic than syngenic CNS and CNS MBP. Of particular interest is the finding that guinea pig CNS preparations and MBP are markedly more encephalitogenic for Lewis rats than syngenic encephalitogens [Paterson et al., 1970; McFarlin et al., 1973].

Other Important Variables

The composition and preparation of the emulsion, the site of injection, and the number of injections can influence the production of EAE. This is particularly true in disease induced in SJL/J mice by the injection of spinal cord homogenate. The species and amount of Mycobacteria was critical. When more than 60 μg was administered suppression of disease was observed in SJL mice [Brown and McFarlin, 1981].

Some investigators use additional adjuvants in order to obtain more intense and/or reproducible disease. *Bordetella pertussis* is widely used for the production of EAE in mice. It is believed that the mode of action is through an effect on vascular permeability [Linthicum and Frelinger, 1982].

Myelin Basic Protein

MBP, a major protein constituent of the myelin membrane, has been known for over three decades to be encephalitogenic and has been extensively investigated. Studies have centered on the biochemical characterization of MBP [Martenson, 1983], identification of disease-causing epitopes within the molecule [Alvord, 1983], the role of genetics in expression of clinical EAE in the experimental animal [Gasser et al., 1973; Webb et al., 1973a, b; Fritz et al., 1985a, b], and most recently, the structure of the MBP gene and its expression [Zeller et al., 1984; DeFerra et al., 1985; Takahashi et al., 1985; Kamholz et al., 1986].

MBP exists as several isoforms that vary in the number and structure in different animal species. For example, five isoforms have been identified in the mouse [Newman et al., 1987] and four in humans [Kamholz et al., 1986; Roth et al., 1987]. The isoforms are derived from a single gene spanning > 30 kb composed of seven exons interrupted by introns of varying size. The gene has been localized to the distal end of chromosome 18 in both the mouse and the human [Roach et al., 1985; Saxe et al., 1985].

The isoforms vary in molecular weight from 14 to 21.5 kilodaltons (kD) and are generated by alternative mRNA splicing mechanisms [DeFerra et al., 1985]. cDNA coding for five isoforms of mouse MBP and four

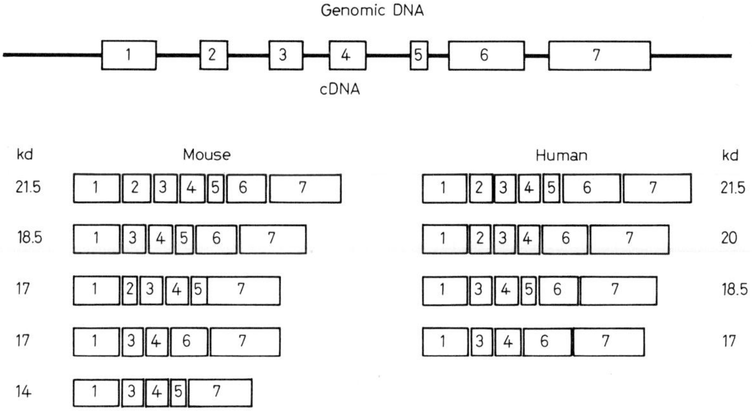

Fig. 2. Structure of the MBP gene and cDNA from mouse and man.

isoforms of human MBP have been isolated (fig. 2). The cDNAs from the mouse code for isoforms of 21.5, 18.5, 17 (2), and 14 kD. The human isoforms are 21.5, 18.5, 17, and 14 kD in size.

In the mouse alternative splicing of exons 2, 5 and 6 accounts for all the mRNA species and resultant isoforms. In the human the four isoforms are derived by alternate splicing of exons 2 and 5 of the primary transcript. It is of interest that the expression of the various isoforms is strictly regulated during development although the mechanism of regulation is not known at present. For example, the ratio of the 14-kD form to the 18.5-kD form in the mouse increases dramatically during development with the result that the two isoforms are expressed at high level in the adult. In the human and a number of other species only the 18.5-kD form is expressed at a high level in the adult. The biological function of each of the isoforms has not been elucidated.

MBP is highly conserved among species [Martenson, 1983]. Amino acid interchanges and deletions at known positions within the molecule have provided valuable information as to the location of regions which carry encephalitogenic epitopes within the MBP molecule (fig. 3). Due to the existence of different isoforms as well as the presence of small deletions with MBP molecules from different species, the numbering system for these molecules is inconsistent and confusing. Among mammals the 18.5-kD form of porcine MBP contains the largest number of amino acids and is used as a reference for numbering of MBP from other species (table 4). This allows the mammalian molecules to be compared directly to each other without compensation for small deletions which occur at different places.

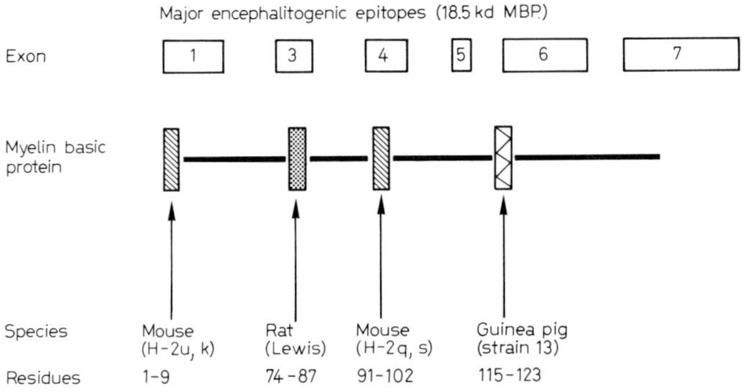

Fig. 3. Regions within the MBP molecule which are major encephalitogenic sites for different species.

When the amino acid sequences of the mammalian MBP are compared, there are no regions of distinct hypervariability. The region coded for by exon 7 is constant from one species to another. The remainder of the molecule has single amino acid interchanges and randomly scattered small deletions throughout the molecule. The deletions are almost always associated with a histidine residue with the majority being His, Gly.

Encephalitogenic Epitopes of Myelin Basic Protein

Although a number of different models of EAE induced in various species of experimental animals by whole CNS tissue have been described, the present discussion will be limited to the results of studies carried out in inbred animals using MBP or enzymatic or synthetic peptides of MBP. A summary of major and minor encephalitogenic MBP eptopes in a variety of outbred and inbred species has been presented previously [Alvord, 1983].

It is significant that there is no single region of the molecule which serves as a general encephalitogen for all species. Different sequences are encephalitogenic for different species (fig. 3, table 5). For example, the sequence 70–90 of guinea pig MBP is highly encephalitogenic for the Lewis rat [McFarlin et al., 1973; Martenson et al., 1975], but is not encephalitogenic for the mouse [Pettinelli et al., 1982; Fritz et al., 1983a]. In mice different regions of the molecule are encephalitogenic for different inbred strains. Residues 1–9 are encephalitogenic for H-2^u mice [Zamvil et al., 1986; Urban et al., 1988] while at least two epitopes (residues 91–102 and 95–108) are encephalitogenic for SJL/J mice [Kono et al., 1988; Sakai et al., 1988]. Guinea pigs respond to residues 114–123 [Eylar and Hashim, 1968; Martenson et al., 1972]. There appears to be no significant sequence

Table 4. Amino acid sequences of MBP of several mammalian species

										10										20										30					
Pig	A	S	Q	K	R	P	S	Q	R	H	G	S	K	Y	L	A	S	A	S	T	M	D	H	A	R	H	G	F	L	P	R	H	R	D	T
Hum	A	S	Q	K	R	P	S	Q	R	H	G	S	K	Y	L	A	T	A	S	T	M	D	H	A	R	H	G	F	L	P	R	H	R	D	T
Chim	A	S	Q	K	R	P	S	Q	R	H	G	S	K	Y	L	A	T	A	S	T	M	D	H	A	R	H	G	F	L	P	R	H	R	D	T
Bov	A	S	Q	K	R	P	S	Q	R	—	—	S	K	Y	L	A	S	A	S	T	M	D	H	A	R	H	G	F	L	P	R	H	R	D	T
Rab	A	S	Q	K	R	P	S	Q	R	H	G	S	K	Y	L	A	T	A	S	T	M	D	H	A	R	H	G	F	L	P	R	H	R	D	T
GP	A	S	Q	K	R	P	S	Q	R	H	G	S	K	Y	L	A	T	A	S	T	M	D	H	A	R	H	G	F	L	P	R	H	R	D	T
Rat	A	S	Q	K	R	P	S	Q	R	H	G	S	K	Y	L	A	T	A	S	T	M	D	H	A	R	H	G	F	L	P	R	H	R	D	T
Mou	A	S	Q	K	R	P	S	Q	R	—	—	S	K	Y	L	A	T	A	S	T	M	D	H	A	R	H	G	F	L	P	R	H	R	D	T

					40										50										60										70
Pig	G	I	L	D	S	L	G	R	F	F	G	A	D	R	G	A	P	K	R	G	S	G	K	D	G	H	H	A	A	R	T	T	H	Y	G
Hum	G	I	L	D	S	L	G	R	F	F	G	G	D	R	G	A	P	K	R	G	S	G	K	D	S	H	H	A	A	R	T	T	H	Y	G
Chim	G	I	L	D	S	L	G	R	F	F	G	G	D	R	G	A	P	K	R	G	S	G	K	D	G	H	H	A	A	R	T	T	H	Y	G
Mon										F	G	G	D	R	G	V	P	K	R	G	S	G	K	D	S	H	H	A	A	R	T	T	H	Y	G
Bov	G	I	L	D	S	L	G	R	F	F	G	S	D	R	G	A	P	K	R	G	S	G	K	D	G	H	H	A	A	R	T	T	H	Y	G
Rab	G	I	L	D	S	L	G	R	F	F	S	S	D	R	G	A	P	K	R	G	S	G	K	D	—	—	H	A	A	R	T	T	H	Y	G
GP	G	I	L	D	S	L	G	R	F	F	G	S	D	R	G	A	P	K	R	G	S	G	K	D	S	H	H	A	A	R	T	T	H	Y	G
Rat	G	I	L	D	S	L	G	R	F	F	S	G	D	R	G	A	P	K	R	G	S	G	K	D	S	H	—	—	T	R	T	T	H	Y	G
Mou	G	I	L	D	S	L	G	R	F	F	S	A	D	R	G	A	P	K	R	G	S	G	K	D	G	H	—	—	T	R	T	T	H	Y	G

										80										90										100					
Pig	S	L	P	Q	K	A	Q	H	G	R	P	Q	D	E	N	P	V	V	H	F	F	K	N	I	V	T	P	R	T	P	P	P	S	Q	G
Hum	S	L	P	Q	K	S	—	H	G	R	T	Q	D	E	N	P	V	V	H	F	F	K	N	I	V	T	P	R	T	P	P	P	S	Q	G
Chim	S	L	P	Q	K	S	—	H	G	R	T	Q	D	E	N	P	V	V	H	F	F	K	N	I	V	T	P	R	T	P	P	P	S	Q	G
Mon	S	L	P	Q	K	S	—	H	G	R	T	Q	D	E	N	P	V	V	H	F															

Bov	S	L	P	Q	K	A	Q	H	G	R	P	Q	D	E	N	P	V	V	H	F	F	K	N	I	V	T	P	R	T	P	P	P	S	Q	G
Rab	S	L	P	Q	K	S	—	H	G	R	P	Q	D	E	N	P	V	V	H	F	F	K	N	I	V	T	P	R	T	P	P	P	S	Q	G
GP	S	L	P	Q	K	S	Q	—	—	R	S	Q	D	E	N	P	V	V	H	F	F	K	N	I	V	T	P	R	T	P	P	P	S	Q	G
Rat	S	L	P	Q	K	S	Q	—	—	R	T	Q	D	E	N	P	V	V	H	F	F	K	N	I	V	T	P	R	T	P	P	P	S	Q	G
Mou	S	L	P	Q	K	S	—	H	G	R	T	Q	D	E	N	P	V	V	H	F	F	K	N	I	V	T	P	R	T	P	P	P	S	Q	G

					110										120										130										140
Pig	K	G	R	G	L	S	L	S	R	F	S	W	G	A	E	G	Q	K	P	G	F	G	Y	G	G	R	A	P	D	Y	K	P	A	H	K
Hum	K	G	R	G	L	S	L	S	R	F	S	W	G	A	E	G	Q	K	P	G	F	G	Y	G	G	R	A	S	D	Y	K	S	A	H	K
Chim	K	G	R	G	L	S	L	S	R	F	S	W	G	A	E	G	Q	K	P	G	F	G	Y	G	G	R	S	P	D	Y	K	S	A	H	K
Mon																																			
Bov	K	G	R	G	L	S	L	S	R	F	S	W	G	A	E	G	Q	K	P	G	F	G	Y	G	G	R	A	S	D	Y	K	S	A	H	K
Rab	K	G	R	G	L	S	L	S	R	F	S	W	G	A	E	G	Q	K	P	G	F	G	Y	G	G	R	A	A	D	Y	K	S	A	H	K
GP	K	G	R	G	L	S	L	S	R	F	S	W	G	A	E	G	Q	K	P	G	F	G	Y	G	G	R	A	—	D	Y	K	S	—	—	K
Rat	K	G	R	G	L	S	L	S	R	F	S	W	G	A	E	G	Q	K	P	G	F	G	Y	G	G	R	A	S	D	Y	K	S	A	H	K
Mou	K	G	R	G	L	S	L	S	R	F	S	W	G	A	E	G	Q	K	P	G	F	G	Y	G	G	R	A	S	D	Y	K	S	A	H	K

										150										160										170		
Pig	G	L	K	G	A	Q	D	A	Q	G	T	L	S	K	I	F	K	L	G	G	R	D	S	R	S	G	S	P	M	A	R	R
Hum	G	L	K	G	V	—	D	A	Q	G	T	L	S	K	I	F	K	L	G	G	R	D	S	R	S	G	S	P	M	A	R	R
Chim	G	L	K	G	A	Q	D	A	Q	G	T	L	S	K	I	F	K	L	G	G	R	D	S	R	S	G	S	P	M	A	R	R
Mon																																
Bov	G	L	K	G	—	H	D	A	Q	G	T	L	S	K	I	F	K	L	G	G	R	D	S	R	S	G	S	P	M	A	R	R
Rab	G	L	K	G	A	—	D	A	Q	G	T	L	S	K	I	F	K	L	G	G	R	D	S	R	S	G	S	P	M	A	R	R
GP	G	L	K	G	A	H	D	A	Q	G	T	L	S	K	I	F	K	L	G	G	R	D	S	R	S	G	S	P	M	A	R	R
Rat	G	L	K	G	A	—	D	A	Q	G	T	L	S	K	I	F	K	L	G	G	R	D	S	R	S	G	S	P	M	A	R	R
Mou	G	L	K	G	A	Y	D	A	Q	G	T	L	S	K	I	F	K	L	G	G	R	D	S	R	S	G	S	P	M	A	R	R

Table 5. Encephalitogenic epitopes for different species of mammals

Species	Residues[a]	Encephalitogenic Sequence
Mouse		
PL/J	1–9	A S Q K R P S Q R
SJL/J	91–102	F K N I V T P R T P P P
SJL/J	95–108	V T P R T P P P S Q G K G R
Rat		
Lewis	71–90	S L P Q K S Q - - R T Q D E N P V V H F
Guinea pig		
Strain 13	115–123	F S W G A E G Q K

[a] Residue number based on the sequence of pig MBP.

similarity between these different epitopes. An important point made by these findings is that encephalitogenic regions for humans are likely to be different from those for other species. Indeed, encephalitogenic regions may vary for different individuals.

An important, but unresolved, issue is raised by the finding of unique encephalitogenic determinants in each species or strain. Possibilities include differences in T cell repertoires, antigen processing, exposure of epitopes in the CNS, or unique Ia-peptide interactions among various species.

The initial event of the encephalitogenic process is the immune response to MBP. As with many antigens, the response to MBP is under IR gene control. Studies of the fine specificity of the T cell reponse to myoglobin, cytochrome *c*, hen egg lysozyme and other antigens have shown that each MHC haplotype responds to a particular spectrum of dominant and subdominant epitopes, and that the spectrum may differ for different haplotypes [Hill and Sercarz, 1975; Barcinski and Rosenthal, 1977; Berzofsky et al, 1977, 1979; Rosenwasser et al., 1979; Hedrick et al., 1982; Matis et al., 1982; Riley et al., 1982; Suzuki and Schwartz, 1986]. The finding of different encephalitogenic epitopes for different species or strains is in accord with an IR under IR gene control.

It has been shown that the MHC controls the specificity of the encephalitogenic response in MHC-congenic mice (table 2). For example, A/J mice (I-A^k) respond to peptide 1–20 while A.SW mice (I-A^s) respond to peptide 91–102. Likewise, B10.PL mice (I-A^u) react against peptide 1–11 whereas B10.T(6R) mice (I-A^q) respond to peptide 91–172 [Fritz et al., 1985a]. Since the T cell antigen receptor repertoire should be identical in MHC-congenic mice on the A- or B10-background, the encephalitogenic specificity is not determined by this property. Additionally, it seems unlikely that there would be different exposure of epitopes on MBP in the CNS or differential antigen processing in MHC-congenic strains.

Current immunological thought would favor the hypothesis that an encephalitogenic epitope is formed by a unique interaction of a MBP peptide with an I-region antigen, I-A^s with peptide 91–103 in the case of SJL mice [Adorini et al., 1988; Lorenz and Allen, 1988]. This would result in a 'dominant' epitope, and that the T cell response would be directed predominantly against this region of the molecule. Likewise, peptide 1–9 would form a unique interaction with I-A^u. This would not preclude other MBP peptides from interaction with I-A^s or I-A^u to form 'subdominant' epitopes or suppressor epitopes.

It has been found that animals immunized with MBP generate significant T cell reactivity, as measured by in vitro lymphocyte proliferative response, against epitopes removed from the encephalitogenic region in addition to strong reactivity against the encephalitogenic epitope [Pettinelli et al., 1982; Fritz et al., 1983a]. T cells directed against the former epitopes (subdominant) are not encephalitogenic when cultured for short periods of time under conditions which favor selection for encephalitogenic activity. For example, Pettinelli et al. [1982] reported that lymph node cells taken from MBP-immune mice would transfer EAE adoptively when cultured in vitro with MBP or peptide 91–172. The same lymph node cells proliferated well to peptide 1–39, but did not transfer disease adoptively. These results show that SJL T cells can react against nonencephalitogenic peptides. However, the activated T cells specific for the latter epitope did not transfer EAE adoptively.

Very recently, Kono et al. [1988] reported that SJL T cell lines obtained from mice immunized with synthetic MBP peptides 91–102 and 95–108 were encephalitogenic. The findings of these workers indicated that each peptide contained an unique epitope. However, these peptides did not react with a T cell line against rat MBP. It was concluded that these peptides represented minor (subdominant) encephalitogenic eptiopes. These data indicate that the SJL mouse recognizes multiple encephalitogenic epitopes.

It has been demonstrated in both the mouse and the rat that only a fraction of the T cell population directed against the encephalitogenic epitope is capable of disease induction [Vandenbark et al., 1985; Acha-Orbea et al., 1988]. Encephalitogenic and nonencephalitogenic T cell clones may have identical fine specificity for the antigen and very similar rearrangements of genes encoding the alpha and beta chains of the T cell antigen receptor [Acha-Orbea et al., 1988; Urban et al., 1988; Zamvil et al., 1988]. Thus, the factors which make a MBP-specific T cell encephalitogenic are unknown at present; however, it is clear that properties intrinsic to the T cell in addition to specific reactivity with an encephalitogenic epitope play critical roles.

Taken together the above findings raise several important questions. First, is the concept a single pathogenic epitope in an autoantigen such as MBP correct? It would seem theoretically possible that any epitope could be encephalitogenic under the proper conditions. What is usually studied is a dominant epitope that induces a strong cellular response. Within the population of T cells responding to the dominant epitope may be a relatively small subpopulation of EAE effector cells. It is possible that subdominant epitopes are not encephalitogenic under usual conditions due to a quantitatively weaker response of the host, and that the responding T cell population contains too few EAE effectors to cause disease. If this concept is correct, it might be possible to expand encephalitogenic T cells against subdominant epitopes during long-term in vitro culture.

It is clear that the antigen-specific T cell receptor is not the sole criterion of encephalitogenicity. Therefore, other biological and biochemical properties of EAE effector T cells may be important in the pathogenesis of EAE. Do the effector cells produce a particular set of lymphokines, do they home to a particular region and interact with the target, or do they require antigen to be presented by a specialized antigen-presenting cell (APC, astrocytes, endothelial cells, microglia)? The answers to these and other questions are critical to understanding the autoimmune process.

An Immune Response Enigma

Many of the early studies of murine EAE were done in SJL strain since this strain was found to show signs of EAE at a relatively high frequency following immunization with CNS tissue emulsified in complete adjuvant. Usually only a fraction of the mice exhibited clinical signs in any given experiment. A similar situation was observed when the mice were immunized with MBP. Subsequently, EAE was produced in other strains, and it was recognized that encephalitogenic epitopes were different. SJL mice were bred with PL/J mice because the two strains responded to different encephalitogenic epitopes (table 2). The F1 hybrid mice were found to be more susceptible ($>90\%$) than either parental strain to clinical EAE and also developed chronic, relapsing disease [Fritz et al., 1983a].

Interestingly, when the F1 hybrid mice were immunized with the encephalitogenic peptides for each strain, the N-terminal peptide, which was encephalitogenic for PL/J mice, caused disease in the large majority of mice [Fritz et al., 1983a]. The C-terminal peptide caused disease in an occasional F1 hybrid. This was the identical immune response phenotype of the PL/J parent. In an attempt to analyze the reason for the observed dominance, in vitro antigen presentation studies were carried out. The ability of SJL/J, PL/J, or F1 hybrid APC to present antigen to MBP-primed purified peritoneal exudate T cells was assessed. Surprisingly, SJL APC presented antigen to F1 T cells poorly although they presented well to SJL T cells [Fritz et al., 1985b]. At the clonal level virtually all antigen-specific T cell clones derived from MBP-immune F1 hybrid mice were restricted to I-A^u or hybrid I-A [Zamvil et al., 1985a, b]. A similar, but less profound effect, was observed in experiments with purified lymph node T cells carried out by McCarron and McFarlin [1988]. Additionally, these workers found that MBP-primed F1 hybrid T cells could adoptively transfer EAE following short-term culture with peptide 89–169 and SJL APC.

The phenomenon of biased presentation was not antigen-specific as a similar effect was observed when ovalbumin was used as the priming antigen [Fritz et al., 1985b]. Comparable findings were obtained with (SWR/J × PL/J)F1 and B10 × PL/J)F1 hybrid mice although in the case of the latter hybrid, the effect was less pronounced. It is significant that SJL, SWR and B10 mice do not express I-E class II molecules [Ozato et al., 1980; Jones et al., 1981; Mathis et al., 1983]. In another experiment A/J mice, which express I-E molecules were crossed with PL/J mice. The (A/J × PL)F1 mice did not show significant unbalanced antigen expression. These findings implicate I-E in this phenomenon.

Further, SJL and SWR have deleted a significant portion of the Vβ genes of the β chain of the T cell antigen receptor [Behlke et al., 1986]. T cell clones from mice of the latter strains have found to be highly reactive against molecules of the I-E subregion [Kappler et al., 1987]. The possibility exists that, during thymic differentiation, T cells which are alloreactive against I-E^u molecules are eliminated. This would lead to a skewing of the T cell populations in (SJL × PL)F1 and (SWR × PL)F1 toward the PL parental type if a significant number of non-PL T cells were eliminated. a similar, but less exterme, effect might occur in (B10 × Pl)F1 hybrid mice.

Alternatively, in view of the findings of McCarron and McFarlin [1988] with lymph node T cells, the observed in vivo bias may be due to active suppression induced by a mechanism which involved the I-E^u molecule. This effect might be less apparent in vitro with lymph node cells and could be overridden during adoptive transfer of activated T cells.

A third possibility is that the bias in these F1 hybrid mice might be due to unbalanced expression of I-A molecules in the F1. However, (SJL × PL)F1 APC present antigen to antigen-specific SJL T cell clones in a normal manner [Zamvil et al., 1985a, b], and two-dimensional gel analysis indicates that I-A^s is present in the F1 in normal amounts [Fritz, unpublished].

Dissection of an Encephalitogenic Peptide

The most complete study of the properties of an encephalitogenic peptide with respect to structure and function was carried out on the disease-inducing determinant for the Lewis rat. Peptide 70–90 of guinea pig MBP is as potent as the intact protein on an equimolar basis [McFarlin et al., 1973]. Immunization with this peptide emulsified in complete Freund's adjuvant results in T cell immunity manifested by EAE in vivo and a lymphoproliferative response in vitro when lymph node cells from immune animals are cultured with either MBP or the peptide. In addition, the same animals develop a vigorous antibody response directed against the peptide [Kibler et al., 1977].

The peptide was then dissected enzymatically in order to identify the epitopes involved in B and T cell reactivity. Residues 79–90 contained an epitope(s) reactive with antibody. This peptide behaved as a classical hapten in that it was reactive with serum antibody, but nonimmunogenic [Fritz et al., 1979]. Peptide 70–87, on the other hand, induced T cell response in vivo and in vitro, but did not react with antibody directed against peptide 70–90. After immunization with peptide 70–87 antibody was produced although it did not react with the 70–89 peptide [Fritz et al., 1979]. When the structures of peptide 70–90 and 70–87 were examined by circular dichroism, it was found that the conformations were different [Fritz et al., 1979]. Thus, the epitopes against which antibody reacted were conformation-dependent whereas the T cell epitope was independent of conformation in agreement with earlier studies with other protein antigens.

The T cell epitope was further defined by two approaches. First, natural variants of the peptide were isolated from rat and bovine MBP. The rat and guinea pig sequence are identical with the exception of a Ser to Thr interchange at position 81 [Chou et al., 1977]. The bovine peptide was a Pro at this position in addition to a Gly-His insertion at positions 78–79. With respect to induction of EAE the guinea pig sequence is approximately 100-fold more active than the rat peptide. A similar difference in activity is seen in vitro. The bovine peptide is virtually inactive. Thus, residue 81 is critical for the T cell epitope.

The second approach was to prepare subpeptides of varying length from peptide 70–90. The shortest peptide which retained full encephalitogenic acitvity was peptide 73–88. All peptides of shorter length showed reduced or no encephalitogenic activity [Chou et al., 1979]. Similar results were reported by Mannie et al. [1985] using synthetic peptides.

In summary, the findings of these studies were (1) the T and B cell epitopes of encephalitogenic peptide 70–90 were distinct, but overlapping; (2) the T cell epitope was insensitive to conformational alterations; (3) the shortest peptide which retained full activity was peptide 73–88; and (4) residue 81 was critical for T cell activity.

Prevention and Suppression of EAE

Because it has been postulated that the pathogenetic mechanisms leading to the production of EAE may also be operative in human demyelinating disease, there has been a longstanding interest in modifying or suppressing the experimental disease. Much work has been done in this area and some of the findings have been extrapolated to therapeutic trials in human disorders.

However, biological mechanisms for the observed phenomenon remain to be clearly defined for at least two reasons. First, the different variables in the production of EAE render it difficult, and perhaps impossible, to extrapolate from one system to another. Second, concepts of immune regulation and suppression remain in evolution and have changed dramatically over the past decade. Also, many of these studies have been carried out in mice and, thus, do not always apply to other species such as guinea pigs and rats.

The studies in EAE can be conveniently grouped into the following areas: (1) treatment with steroids and immune suppressants; (2) prevention of EAE by preimmunization with encephalitogen in incomplete adjuvant; (3) immunization with synthetic polypeptides; (4) suppressor cells; and (5) treatment with antibodies to T cells and/or MHC antigens.

Areas 2, 3 and 4 relate directly to the concepts covered in this article and will be discussed in more detail.

Prevention by Preimmunization with Encephalitogen

Immunization with MBP in *incomplete* adjuvant leads to suppression of clinical EAE upon subsequent challenge with MBP in *complete* adjuvant. If such a regimen were used for the treatment of patients, it would be advantageous if nonencephalitogenic material were to be used for immunization. The encephalitogenic determinant for guinea pigs is contained within residues 114–123 of bovine MBP and tryptophan at position 117 is essential. Swanborg [1972] modified this residue with 2-hydroxy-5-nitrobenzenebromide and rendered the protein nonencephalitogenic. Immunization with the modified protein protected guinea pigs from subsequent challenge with unmodified protein. Later, the same laboratory reported that nonencephalitogenic peptide 45–90 of bovine MBP protected against challenge with intact protein [Swanborg, 1975]. The implication of the work was that peptide 45–90 contained suppressor epitopes.

Later Driscoll et al. [1976] reported that only the encephalitogenic fragment of MBP would protect guinea pigs from challenge with intact protein. However, the fragment used for protection consisted of residues 92–172 which could have contained a suppressor epitope in addition to the encephalitogenic epitope.

In order to clarify this issue, Kibler and colleagues [Chou et al., 1980] carried out a study on the protective effects of guinea pig encephalitogenic peptide 70–90 emulsified in incomplete adjuvant from the rat, guinea pig and cow were injected into rats. After a period of weeks the animals were challenged with guinea pig peptide 70–90. As little as 0.02 μg of the guinea pig peptide afforded a significant degree of protection. A 1,000-fold higher dose of rat peptide afforded no protection.

When truncated peptides derived form peptide 70–90 were tested, the protective effect exactly paralleled their encephalitogenic activity when administered in complete adjuvant. Peptide 70–90 was most protective followed by peptide 70–87 and 70–86. All other peptides tested were ineffective. The conclusion derived from this set of experiments was that only encephalitogenic peptides were effective for protection. The applicability of these findings to other experimental systems, particularly in different species, remains to be demonstrated.

Preimmunization with Synthetic Polypeptides

During studies of the encephalitogenic epitope in guinea pigs specific amino acids essential for disease induction were identified. This led to the concept that synthetic polypeptides which simulated MBP in size and charge might suppress disease. A series of such polypeptides was produced and tested. The most widely studied of these polypeptides is Cop I, a random copolymer of *L*-alanine, *L*-glutamic acid, *L*-Lysine, and *L*-tyrosine in the ratio of 6.0:1.9:4.7:1.0 and molecular weight of 1,4000–23,000 daltons. Treatment of guinea pigs with Cop I suppresses EAE both clinically and histologically. Apparently, suppression is not epitope-specific since this polypeptide also suppresses the disease in rabbits, subhuman primates and mice [Teitelbaum et al., 1971, 1973, 1974; Keith et al., 1979].

The possibility that Cop I was a general immunosuppressant was considered, but no effect on formation of antibody to BSA, RNAase, DNP, or T4 bacteriophage was observed. Guinea pigs treated with Cop I developed DTH to both Cop I and MBP, but not to lysozyme, another basic protein [Webb et al., 1973a, b, 1976]. Less cross-reactivity was detected between Cop I and MBP with lymphocyte proliferative response. On the basis of these findings it was postulated that suppressive effects were due to cross-reactivity of MBP and Cop I. The mechanism of suppression was postulated to be through suppressor T cells.

Suppressor Cells

Although the events responsible for the pathogenesis of EAE are not fully understood, it is likely that endogenous regulatory mechanisms are operative. In rats EAE is monophasic and following recovery from the acute episode, additional immunizations do not lead to disease. This appears to be an active process because it can be abolished by total body irradiation [Willenborg, 1979] or the administration of cyclophosphamide [Miyazaki et al., 1985]. Resistance can be transferred to syngeneic naive recipients by T cells. The recipients were not protected from adoptively transferred EAE, however, which indicated that the suppressive effect was manifested during the inductive phase of the encephalitogenic response [Sweirkosz and Swanborg, 1975; Welch and Swanborg, 1976; Willenborg, 1979].

Recently T cell lines that down-regulate EAE in the rat have been described. A $CD4^+$ cell line selected in the presence of ciclosporin A blocks the capacity of encephalitogenic T cell to transfer disease adoptively following in vitro co-culture of the lines [Ellerman et al., 1988]. In another study a $CD8^+$ cell line that blocks the transfer of EAE and has specificity for the encephalitogenic T cell line was described [Sun et al., 1988]. The implication from both studies is that similar mechanisms operate in vivo.

In mice preimmunization with MBP in incomplete adjuvant blocks production of EAE. Suppression can be transferred with spleen cells. Administration of MBP coupled to spleen cells also induced protection from subsequent challenge Sriram et al. [1983]. Other evidence for the existence of suppressor cells is reviewed by Arnon [1981].

Conclusions

In recent years considerable progress has been made in understanding T-cell-mediated CNS disease. This has paralleled advances in fundamental immunology. However, in spite of this progress, several unresolved questions remain. The first concerns the generation of and properties of EAE effector T cells, and whether these are directed against a single pathogenic epitope on the encephalitogenic molecule.

A second unresolved area concerns the mechanisms which lead to T-cell-mediated tissue damage. How do the effector cells reach the CNS? What cells within the CNS present antigen to the effectors? What is their target, and by what mechanism do they damage the target?

A third important area is that of regulation of the immune response leading to disease. Does regulation operate at the level of T cell differentiation, or in the target tissue? At the rate at which immunology is progressing, it should not be too many years before we know the answers to these questions.

References

Acha-Orbea, H.; Mitchell, D.; Timmermann, L.; Wratih, D.; Tausch, G.; Waldor, M.; Zamvil, S.; McDevitt, H.; Steinman, L.: Limited heterogeneity of T cell receptors from lymphocytes mediating autoimmune encephalomyelitis allows specific immune intervention. Cell *54:* 263 (1988).

Adorini, L.; Sette, A.; Buus, S.; Grey, H.; Darsley, M.; Lehmann, P.; Doria, G.; Nagy, Z.; Appella, E.: Interaction of an immunodominant epitope with Ia molecules in T-cell activation. Proc. natn. Acad. Aci. USA *85:* 5181 (1988).

Alvord, E.C., Jr.: Species-restricted encephalitogenic determinants. Prog. clin. biol. Res. *146:* 523 (1983).

Arnon, R.: Experimental allergic encephalomyelitis – susceptibility and suppression. Immunol. Rev. *55:* 5 (1981).

Barcinski, M.; Rosenthal, A.S.: Immune response gene control of determinant selection. I. Intramolecular mapping of the immunogenic sites on insullin recognized by guinea pig T and B cells. J. exp. Med. *145:* 726 (1977).

Behlke, M.; Chou, H.; Huppi, K.; Loh, D.: Murine T cell receptor mutants with deletions of beta-chain variable region genes. Proc. natn. Acad. Sci. USA *83:* 767 (1986).

Ben-Nun, A.; Lando, Z.: Detection of autoimmmune cells proliferating to myelin basic protein and selection of T cell lines that mediate experimental allergic encephalomyelitis (EAE) in mice. J. Immun. *130:* 1205 (1983).

Ben-Nun, A.; Otmy, H.; Cohen, I.: Genetic control of autoimmune encephalomyelitis and recognition of the critical nonapeptide moiety of myelin basic protein are exerted through interaction of lymphocytes and macrophages. Eur. J. Immunol. *11:* 311 (1981a).

Ben-Nun, A.; Wekerle, H.; Cohen, I.: The rapid isolation of clonable antigen-specific T lymphocyte lines capable of mediating autoimmune encephalomyelitis. Eur. J. Immunol. *11:* 195 (1981b).

Bernard, C.: Experimental autoimmune encephalomyelitis in mice: genetic control of susceptibility. J. Immunogenet. *3:* 263 (1976).

Berzofsky, J.A.; Richman, L.K.; Killion, D.J.: Distinct H-2-linked Ir genes control both antibody and T cell responses to different determinants on the same antigen, myoglobin. Proc. natn. Acad. Sci. USA *76:* 4046 (1979).

Berzofsky, J.A.; Schecter, A.N.; Shearer, G.M.; Sachs, D.H.: Genetic control of the immune response to Staphyloccal nuclease. IV. H-2-linked control of the relative proportions of antibodies produced to different determinants of native nuclease. J. exp. Med. *145:* 123 (1977).

Brown, A.; McFarlin, D.E.: Relapsing experimental allergic encephalomyelitis in the SJL/J mouse. Lab. Invest. *45:* 278 (1981).

Chou, C.-H.J.; Chou, F.C.-H.; Kowalski, T.; Shapira, R.; Kibler, R.: The major site of guinea pig myelin basic protein in Lewis rats. J. Neurochem. *28:* 115 (1977).

Chou, C.-H.J.; Fritz, R.; Chou, F.C.-H.; Kibler, R.: The immune response of Lewis rats to peptide 68–88 of guinea pig myelin basic protein. I. T cell determinants. J. Immun. *123:* 1540 (1979).

Chou, F.C-H.; Chou, C.-H.J.; Fritz, R.; Kibler, R.: Prevention of experimental allergic encephalomyelitis in Lewis rats with peptide 68–88 of guinea pig myelin basic protein. Ann. Neurol. *7:* 336 (1980).

DeFerra, F.; Engh, H.; Hudson, L; Kamholz, J; Puckett, C.; Molineaux, S.; Lazzarini, R.: Alternative splicing accounts for the four forms of myelin basic protein. Cell *43:* 721 (1985).

Driscoll, B.; Kies, M.; Alvord, E., Jr.: Protection against experimental allergic encephalomyelitis with peptides derived from myelin basic protein: presence of intact encephalitogenic site is essential. J. Immun. *117:* 110 (1976).

Driscoll, B.; Kies, M.; Alvord, E., Jr.: Transfer of experimental allergic encephalomyelitis with guinea pig peritoneal exudate cells. Science *203:* 547 (1979).

Ellerman, K.E.; Powers, J.M.; Brostoff, S.: A suppressor T-lymphocyte cell line for autoimmune encephalomyelitis. Nature *331:* 265 (1988).

Eylar, E.; Hashim, G.: Allergic encephalomyelitis. The structure of the encephalitogenic determinant. Proc. natn. Acad. Sci. USA *61:* 644 (1968).

Fritz, R.; Chou, F.C.-H.; Chou, C.-H.J.; Kibler, R.: The immune response of Lewis rats to peptide 68–88 of guinea pig myelin basic protein. II. B cell determinants. J. Immun. *123:* 1544 (1979).

Fritz, R.; Chou, C.-H.J.; McFarlin, D.: Induction of experimental allergic encephalomyelitis in PL/J and (SJL/J × PL/J)F1 mice by myelin basic protein and its peptides: localization of a second encephalitogenic determinant. J. Immun. *130:* 191 (1983a).

Fritz, R.; Chou, C.-H.J.; McFarlin, D.: Relapsing murine experimental allergic encephalomyelitis induced by myelin basic protein. J. Immun. *130:* 1024 (1983b).

Fritz, R.; Perry, L.; Chou, C.-H.J.: Genetic control of myelin basic protein-induced experimental allergic encephalomyelitis in mice. Prog. clin. biol. Res. *146:* 235 (1983c).

Fritz, R.B.; Skeen, M.J.; Chou, C.-H.J.; Garcia, M.; Egorov, I.K.: Major histocompatibility complex-linked control of the murine immune response to myelin basic protein. J. Immun. *134:* 2328 (1985a).

Fritz, R.B.; Skeen, M.J.; Ziegler, H.K.: Influence of the $H\text{-}2^u$ haplotype on immune function in F1 hybrid mice. I. Antigen presentation. J. Immun. *134:* 3574 (1985b).

Gasser, D.; Newlin, C.; Palm, J.; Gonatas, N.: Genetic control of susceptibility to experimental allergic encephalomyelitis in rats.

Gonzalez, J.: Un caso de rabia paralitica producida por las inoculaciones preventivas. Gast. Med. Catal. (1988).

Hedrick, S.; Matis, L.; Hecht, T.; Samelson, L; Heber-Katz, E.; Schwartz, R.: The fine specificity of antigen and Ia determinant recognition by T cell hybridoma clones specific for pigeon cytochrome c. Cell *30:* 141 (1982).

Hill, S.W.; Sercarz, E.E.: Fine specificity of the H-2 linked immune response gene for the gallinaceous lysozymes. Eur. J. Immunol. *5:* 317 (1975).

Holda, J.; Swanborg, R.: Autoimmune effector cells. II. Transfer of experimental allergic encephalomyelitis with a subset of T lymphocytes. Eur. J. Immunol. *12:* 453 (1982).

Jones, P.; Murphy, S.; McDevitt, H.: Variable synthesis and expression of E_{alpha} and A_e (E_{beta}) Ia polypeptide chains in mice of different H-2 haplotypes. Immunogenetics *12:* 321 (1981).

Kabat, E.A.; Wolf, A.; Bezer, A.E.: The rapid production of acute disseminated encephalomyelitis in Rhesus monkeys by injection of heterologous and homologous brain tissue with adjuvants. J. exp. Med. *85:* 117 (1947).

Kamholz, J.; Deferra, F.; Puckett, C.; Lazzarini, R.: Identification of three forms of human myelin basic protein by cDNA cloning. Proc. natn. Acad. Sci. USA *83:* 4962 (1986).

Kappler, J.; Wade, T.; White, J.; Kushnir, E.; Blackman, M.; Bill, J.; Roehm, N.; Marrack, P.: A T cell receptor V_{beta} segment that imparts reactivity to a class II major histocompatibility complex product. Cell *49:* 263 (1987).

Keith, A.; Arnon, R.; Teitelbaum, D.; Caspary, E.A.; Wisniewski, H.: The effect of Cop I, a synthetic polypeptide, on chronic relapsing experimental allergic encephalomyelitis in guinea pigs. J. neurol. Sci. *42:* 267 (1979).

Kibler, R.; Fritz, R.; Chou, F.-C.H.; Chou, C.-H.J.; Peacocke, N.; Brown, N.; McFarlin, D.: Immune response of Lewis rats to peptide C1 (residues 68–88) of guinea pig and rat myelin basic proteins. J. exp. Med. *146:* 1323 (1977).

Kies, M.: Chemical studies on an encephalitogenic protein from guinea pig brain. Ann. N.Y. Acad. Sci. *122:* 161 (1965).

Kono, D.; Urban, J.; Horvath, S.; Ando, D.; Saavedra, R.; Hood, L.: Two minor determinants of myelin basic protein in duce experimental allergic encephalomyelitis in SJL/J mice. J. exp. Med. *168:* 213 (1988).

Laatsch, R.; Kies, M.; Gordon, S.; Alvord, E., Jr.: The encephalitogenic activity of myelin isolated by ultracentrifugation. J. exp. Med. *115:* 777 (1962).

Lando, Z.; Teitelbaum, D.; Arnon, R.: Genetic control of susceptibility to experimental allergic encephalomyelitis in mice. Immunogenetics *9:* 435 (1979).

Lemire, M.; Jaques, W.; Weigle, W.: Passive transfer of experimental allergic encephalomyelitis by myelin basic proterin specific $L3T4^{+}$ T cell clones possessing several functions. J. Immun. *137:* 3169 (1986).

Levine, S.; Sowinski, R.: Experimental allergic encephalomyelitis in inbred and outbred mice. J. Immun. *110:* 139 (1973).

Levine, S.; Sowinski, R.: Allergic encephalomyelitis in the reputedly resistant Brown Norway strain of rats. J. Immun. *114:* 597 (1975).

Linthicum, D.; Frelinger, J.: Acute autoimmune encephalomyelitis in mice. II. Susceptibility is controlled by the combination of H-2 and histamine sensitization genes. J. exp. Med. *156:* 31 (1982).

Lorenz, R.; Allen, P.: Direct evidence for functional self-protein/Ia-molecule complexes in vivo. Proc. natn. Acad. Sci. USA *85:* 5220 (1988).

Mannie, M.D.; Paterson, P.Y.; U'Prichard, D.C.; Flouret, G.: Induction of experimental allergic encephalomyelitis in Lewis rats with purified synthetic peptides: delineation of antigenic determinants for encephalitogenicity, in vitro activation of cellular transfer, and proliferation of lymphocytes. Proc. natn. Acad. Sci. USA *82:* 5515 (1985).

Martenson, R.: Myelin basic protein speciation. Prog. clin. biol. Res. *146:* 511 (1983).

Martenson, R.; Deibler, G.; Kies, M.; Levine, S.; Alvord, E., Jr.: Myelin basic proteins of mammalian and submammalian vertebrates: encephalitogenic activities in guinea pigs and rats. J. Immun. *109:* 262 (1972).

Martenson, R.; Levine, S.; Sowinski, R.: The location of regions in guinea pig and bovine myelin basic protein which induce experimental allergic encephalomyelitis in Lewis rats. J. Immun. *114:* 592 (1975).

Mathis, D.; Benoist, C.; Williams, V, II; Kanter, M.; McDevitt, H.: Several mechanisms can account for defective E_{alpha} gene expression in different mouse haplotypes. Proc. natn. Acad. Sci. USA *80:* 273 (1983).

Matis, L.A.; Hedrick, S.M.; Hannum, C.; Ultee, M.E.; Lebwohl, D.; Margoliash, E.; Solinger, A.M.; Lerner, E.A.; Schwartz, R.H.: The T lymphocyte response to cytochrome c. III. Relationship of fine specificity of antigen recognition to major histocompatibility complex genotype. J. Immun. *128:* 2439 (1982).

McCarron, R.; McFarlin, D.: Adoptively transferred experimental allergic encephalomyelitis in SJL/J, PL/J and (SJL/J × PL/J)F1 mice. Influence of I-A haplotype on encephalitogenic epitope of myelin basic protein. J. Immun. *141:* 1143 (1988).

McFarlin, D.; Blank, E.; Kibler, R.; McKneally, S.; Shapira, R.: Experimental allergic encephalomyelitis in the rat: response to encephalitogenic proteins and peptides. Science *179:* 478 (1973).

Miyazaki, C.; Nakamura, T.; Kanako, K.; Ryoichi, M.; Shibasaki, H.: Reintroduction of experimental allergic encephalomyelitis in convalescent rats with cyclophosphamide. J. neurol. Sci. *67:* 277 (1985).

Montgomery, I.; Rauch, H.: Experimental allergic encephalomyelitis (EAE) in mice: primary control of EAE susceptibility is outside of the H-2 complex. J. Immun. *128:* 421 (1982).

Morgan, I.: Allergic encephalomyelitis in monkeys in response to injection of normal monkey tissue. J. exp. Med. *85:* 131 (1947).

Newman, S.; Kitamura, K.; Campagnoni, A.: Identification of a cDNA coding for a fifth form of myelin basic protein in the mouse. Proc. natn. Acad. Sci. USA *84:* 886 (1987).

Ozato, K.; Lunney, J.K.; El Gamil, M.; Sachs, D.: Evidence for the absence of I-E/C antigen expression on the cell surface in mice of the $H\text{-}2^b$ or $H\text{-}2^s$ haplotypes. J. Immun. *125:* 940 (1980).

Panitch, H.; McFarlin, D.: Experimental allergic encephalomyelitis: enhancement of cell-mediated transfer by Concanavalin A. J. Immun. *119:* 1134 (1977).

Paterson, P.: Transfer of allergic encephalomyelitis in rats by means of lymph node cells. J. exp. Med. *111:* 119 (1960).

Patterson, P.; Drobis, O.; Hanson, M; Jacobs, A.: Induction of experimental allergic encephalomyelitis in Lewis rats. Int. Archs Allergy appl. Immunol. *37:* 26 (1970).

Pettinelli, C.; Fritz, R.; Chou, C.-H.J.; McFarlin, D.: Encephalitogenic activity of myelin basic protein in the SJL mouse. J. Immun. *129:* 1209 (1982).

Pettinelli, C.; McFarlin, D.: Adoptive transfer of experimental allergic encephalomyelitis in SJL/J mice after in vitro activation of lymph node cells by myelin basic protein. Requirement for $Lyt1^+2^-$ T lymphocytes. J. Immun. *127:* 1420 (1981).

Raine, C.; Barnett, L.; Brown, A.; Behar, T.; McFarlin, D.: Neuropathology of experimental allergic encephalomyelitis in inbred strains of mice. Lab. Invest. *43:* 150 (1980).

Remlinger, P.: Accidents paralytiques au cours du traitement antirabique. Ann. Inst. Pasteur *625:* (1905).

Richert, J.; Driscoll, B.; Kies, M.; Alvord, E., Jr.: Adoptive transfer of experimental allergic encephalomyelitis: incubation of rat spleen cells with specific antigen. J. Immun. *122:* (1979).

Richert, J.; Lehky, T.; Muehl, L.; Mingioli, E.; McFarlin, D.: Myelin basic protein-specific T cell lines and clones derived from SJL/J mice with experimental allergic encephalomyelitis. J. Neuroimmunol. *8:* 129 (1985).

Riley, R.L.; Wilson, L.D.; Germain, R.N.; Benjamin, D.C.: Immune responses to complex protein antigens. I. MHC control of immune responses to bovine albumin. J. Immun. *129:* 1553 (1982).

Rivers, T.; Sprunt, D.; Berry, G.: Observations on attempts to produce acute disseminated encephalomyelitis in monkeys. J. exp. Med. *58:* 39 (1933).

Roach, A.; Takahashi, N.; Pravtcheva, D.; Ruddle, F.; Hood, L.: Chromosomal mapping of mouse myelin basic protein gene structure and transcription of the partially deleted gene in shiverer mutant mice. Cell *42:* 149 (1985).

Rosenwasser, L.J.; Barcinski, M.; Schwartz, R.H.; Rosenthal, A.S.: Immune response gene control of determinant selection. II. Genetic control of the murine T lymphocyte proliferative response to insulin. J. Immun. *123:* 471 (1979).

Roth, H.; Kronquist, K.; Kerlero-deRosha, N.; Crandall, B.; Campagnoni, A.: Evidence for the expression of four myelin basic protein variants in the developing human spinal cord through cDNA cloning. J. Neurosci. Res. *17:* 321 (1987).

Sakai, K.; Namikawa, T.; Kunishita, T.; Yamanouchi, K.; Tabira, T.: Studies of experimental allergic encephalomyelitis by using encephalitogenic T cell line and clones in euthymic and athymic mice. J. Immun. *137:* 1527 (1986).

Sakai, K.; Zamvil, S.; Mitchell, D.; Lim, M.; Rothbard, J.; Steinman, L.: Characterization of a major encephalitogenic T cell eptiope in SJL/J mice with synthetic oligopeptides of myelin basic protein. J. Neuroimmunol. *19:* 21 (1988).

Satoh, J.; Sakai, K.; Endoh, M.; Koike, F.; Kunishita, T.; Namikawa, T.; Yamamura, T.; Tabira, T.: Experimental allergic encephalomyelitis mediated by murine encephalitogenic cell lines specific for myelin proteolipid apoprotein. J. Immun. *138:* 179 (1987).

Saxe, D.; Takahashi, N.; Hood, L.; Simon, M.: Localization of the human myelin basic protein gene (MBP) to region 18q22 qter by in situ hybridization. Cytogenet. Cell Genet. *39:* 246 (1985).

Sriram, S.; Schwartz, G.; Steinman, L.: Administration of myelin basic protein-coupled spleen cells prevents experimental allergic encephalomyelitis. Cell. Immunol. *75:* 378 (1983).

Stone, S.H.: Transfer of allergic encephalomyelitis by lymph node cells in inbred guinea pigs. Science *134:* 619 (1961).

Stuart, G.; Krikorian, K.: The neuro-paralytic accidents of antirabies treatment. Ann. trop. Med. *22:* 327 (1928).

Sun, D.; Qin, Y.; Chluba, J.; Epplen, J.T.; Wekerle, H.: Suppression of experimentally induced autoimmune encephalomyelitis by cytotoxic T-T interactions. Nature *322:* 843 (1988).

Suzuki, G.; Schwartz, R.H.: The pigeon cytochrome c-specific T cell response of low responder mice. I. Identification of antigenic determinants on fragment 1 to 65. J. Immun. *136:* 230–239 (1986).

Swanborg, R.: Antigen-induced inhibition of experimental allergic encephalomyelitis. I. Inhibition in guinea pigs injected with nonencephalitogenic modified myelin basic protein. J. Immun. *109:* 540 (1972).

Swanborg, R.: Antigen-induced inhibition of experimental allergic encephalomyelitis. III. Localization of an inhibitory site distinct from the major encephalitogenic determinant of myelin basic protein. J. Immun. *114:* 191 (1975).

Sweirkosz, J.; Swanborg, R.: Suppressor cell control of unresponsiveness to experimental allergic encephalomyelitis. J. Immun. *115:* 631 (1975).

Takahashi, N.; Roach, A.; Teplow, D.; Prusiner, S.; Hood, L.: Cloning and characterization of the myelin basic protein gene from the mouse: one gene can encode both 14 kd and 18.5 kd MBPs by alternate use of exons. Cell *42:* 139 (1985).

Teitelbaum, D.; Meshorer, A.; Hirshfeld, T.; Arnon, R.; Sela, M.: Suppression of experimental allergic encephalomyelitis by a synthetic polypeptide. Eur. J. Immunol. *1:* 242 (1971).

Teitelbaum, D.; Webb, C.; Arnon, R.; Sela, M.: Strain differences in susceptibility to experimental allergic encephalomyelitis and the immune response to the encephalitogenic determinant in inbred guinea pigs. Cell. Immunol. *29:* 265 (1977).

Teitelbaum, D.; Webb, C.; Bree, M.; Meshorer, A.; Arnon, R.; Sela, M.: Suppression of experimental allergic encephalomyelitis in rhesus monkeys by a synthetic basic copolymer. Clin. Immunol. Immunopath. *3:* 256 (1974).

Teitelbaum, D.; Webb, C.; Meshorer, A.; Arnon, R.; Sela, M.: Suppression by several synthetic polypeptides of experimental allergic encephalomyelitis in guinea pigs and rabbits with bovine and human basic encephalitogen. Eur. J. Immunol. *3:* 273. (1973).

Trotter, J.; Clark, H.; Collins, K.; Wegescheide, C.; Scarpellini, J.: Myelin proteolipid protein induces demyelinating disease in mice. J. neurol. Sci. *79:* 173 (1987).

Tuohy, V.; Lu, Z.; Sobel, R.; Laursen, R.; Lees, M.: A synthetic peptide from myelin proteolipid protein induces experimental allergic encephalomyelitis. J. Immunol. *141:* 1126 (1988).

Urban, J.; Kumar, V.; Kono, D.; Gomez, C.; Horvath, S.; Clayton, J.; Ando, D.; Sercarz, E.; Hood, L.: Restricted use of T cell receptor V genes in murine autoimmune encephalomyelitis raises possibility for antibody therapy. Cell *54:* 577 (1988).

Vandenbark, A.A.; Gill, T.; Offner, H.: A myelin basic protein-specific T lymphocyte line that mediates experimental autoimmune encephalomyelitis. J. Immun. *135:* 223 (1985).

Waksman, B.; Morrison, L.: Tuberculin type sensitivity to spinal cord antigen in rabbits with isoallergic encephalomyelitis. J. Immun. *66:* 421 (1951).

Webb, C.; Teitelbaum, D.; Arnon, R.; Sela, M.: In vivo and in vitro immunological cross-reactions between basic encephalitogen and synthetic basic polypeptides capable of suppressing experimental allergic encephalomyelitis. Eur. J. Immunol. *3:* 279 (1973a).

Webb, C.; Teitelbaum, D.; Arnon, R.; Sela, M.: Correlation between strain differences in susceptibility to experimental allergic encephalomyelitis and the immune response to encephalitogenic protein in inbred guinea pigs. Immunol. Comm. *2:* 185 (1973b).

Webb, C.; Teitelbaum, D.; Herz, A.; Arnon, R.; Sela, M.: Molecular requirements involved in suppression of EAE by synthetic basic copolymers of amino acids. Immunochemistry *13:* 333 (1976).

Welch, A.; Swanborg, R.: Charaterization of suppressor cells involved in regulation of experimental allergic encephalomyelitis. Eur. J. Immunol. *6:* 910 (1976).

Willenborg, D.O.: Experimental allergic encephalomyelitis in the Lewis rat. Studies on the mechanism of recovery from the disease and acquired resistance to induction. J. Immun. *123:* 1145 (1979).

Williams, R.; Moore, M.: Linkage of susceptibility to experimental allergic encephalomyelitis to the major histocompatibility locus in the rat. J. exp. Med. *138:* 775 (1973).

Witebsky, E.; Steinfeld, J.: Untersuchen über spezifische Antigen-Funktionen von Organen. Z. Immunitatsforsch. *58:* 271 (1928).

Yamamura, T.; Namikawa, T.; Endoh, M.; Kunishita, T.; Tabira, T.: Experimental allergic encephalomyelitis induced by proteolipid apoprotein in Lewis rats. J. Neuroimmunol. *12:* 143 (1986).

Yasuda, T.; Tsumita, T.; Nagai, Y.; Mitsuzawa, E.; Ohtani, S.: Experimental allergic encephalomyelitis in mice. I. Induction of EAE with mouse spinal cord homogenate and myelin basic protein. Jap. J. exp. Med. *45:* 423 (1975).

Zamvil, S.; Mitchell, D.; Lee, N.; Moore, A.; Waldor, M; Sakai, K.; Rothbard, J.; McDevitt, H.; Steinman, L; Acha-Orbea, H.: Predominant expression of a T cell receptor V_{beta} gene subfamily in autoimmune encephalomyelitis. J. exp. Med. *167:* 1586 (1988).

Zamvil, S.; Mitchell, D.; Moore, A.; Kitamura, K.; Steinman, L.; Rothbard, J.: T-cell epitope of the autoantigen myelin basic protein that induces encephalomelitis. Nature *324:* 58 (1986).

Zamvil, S.S.; Nelson, P.A.; Mitchell, D.J.; Knobler, R.L.; Fritz, R.B.; Steinman, L.: Encephalitogenic T cell clones specific for myelin basic protein. An unusual bias in antigen recognition. J. exp. Med. *162:* 2107 (1985a).

Zamvil, S.; Nelson, P.; Trotter, J.; Mitchell, D.; Knobler, R.; Fritz, R.; Steinman, L.: T-cell clones specific for myelin basic protein induce chronic relapsing paralysis and demyelination. Nature *355:* (1985b).

Zeller, N.; Hunkeler, M; Campagnoni, A.; Sprague, J.; Lazzarini, R.: Characterization of mouse myelin basic protein messenger RNAs with a myelin basic protein cDNA clone. Proc. natn. Acad. Sci. USA *81:* 18 (1984).

Robert B. Fritz, PhD, Department of Microbiology and Immunology,
Emory University, Atlanta, GA 30322 (USA)

Sercarz E (ed): Antigenic Determinants and Immune Regulation. Chem Immunol.
Basel, Karger, 1989, vol 46, pp 126–156

Molecular Aspects of Ligand Interaction with Somatic and Immune Receptors: Insights from Studies of the Mammalian Reoviruses

Jeffrey A. Cohen[a], *William V. Williams*[b], *David B. Weiner*[c], *Mark I. Greene*[c]

[a]Departments of Neurology, [b]Medicine, and [c]Pathology and Laboratory Medicine, University of Pennsylvania, Philadelphia, Pa., USA

Introduction

The specificity of the immune response in higher organisms involves the high affinity binding of antigen to receptors on B and T lymphocytes. Both qualitative and quantitative aspects of this response are regulated by soluble factors, whose actions are mediated via interaction with cell surface receptor systems. Some of these factors and their receptors are unique to the immune system. Some are involved in the regulation of growth or function of cells of other tissues.

Viral pathogens represent important targets of the immune system. Recognition of viral components by lymphoid receptors initiates a cascade of immune effector mechanisms. The pathogenesis of viral infection is complex and may lead to alteration of target cell growth via a variety of mechanisms including both direct and indirect effects on both immune and somatic cell receptors.

This article reviews the molecular aspects of the interaction of the mammalian reoviruses with receptors of both somatic tissues and the immune system in the context of the idiotypic network paradigm. Much of our current understanding of reovirus biology is based on the conceptual constructs of the idiotypic network theory and their practical application. The interaction of reoviruses with somatic tissues and cells of the immune system of the host organism is mediated by the viral σ_1 cell attachment protein. 'Ligand-like' anti-receptor antibodies generated experimentally as anti-idiotypes, which react with 'receptor-like' anti-σ_1 antibodies, have been utilized to characterize the structural and functional aspects of reovirus-receptor interaction at a molecular level. Studies of the mammalian reoviruses also have been useful in clarifying the interaction of idiotype with anti-idiotype, idiotypic regulation of immune function, and the potential pathogenetic significance of immune mechanisms related to the idiotypic network.

The Idiotypic Network

Numerous studies, including work in the mammalian reovirus system, have substantiated most aspects of the idiotypic network model [57, 67, 91]. This model predicts that the hypervariable regions of lymphoid receptors express antigenic determinants recognized by other antigen receptors within an animal's immune repertoire. The unique collection of epitopes (idiotopes) which characterize an antibody or lymphoid receptor comprise its idiotype. The antibodies reactive with those idiotopes are known as anti-idiotypes. A large number of both xenogeneic and syngeneic anti-idiotypic antibodies have been generated by the immunization of experimental animals with idiotype. In addition, anti-idiotypic antibodies have been demonstrated to arise as normal constituents of the immune response to a variety of antigens including insulin [97, 111, 114], Bis Q (a nicotinic acetylcholine receptor ligand) [16], tetanus toxoid [46, 102], GM1 ganglioside [74], measles virus [66], alprenolol (a β-adrenergic receptor ligand) [103], glucagon [97], and vasopressin [97].

Included in the antigenic determinants of the idiotype is the antigen-binding site. The interaction of anti-idiotype with this idiotope may mimic the interaction with antigen. Anti-idiotypic antibodies of this class represent internal images of the external antigen and may function as immunologic mimics of the nominal antigen. Anti-idiotypic antibodies have been shown to induce both B and/or T cell-mediated immunity to a number of antigens including reovirus [44, 108, 110], *Streptococcus pneumoniae* [26], lysozyme [50], azobenzenearsonate [124], and *Mycobacterium tuberculosis* [95]. The ability of internal image anti-idiotype antibodies to induce humoral and cellular immunity to the nominal antigen suggests a potential use in vaccines. Investigators have tested such vaccines against a variety of microbial pathogens and neoplasms (table 1).

As for other antigens, the route of immunization and the dose and nature of the immunogen determine the character of the immune response generated [25, 83]. Under certain conditions immunization with anti-idiotype induces humoral immunity [26, 44], T cell-mediated cytotoxicity (T_C) [31, 110], delayed-type hypersensitivity (DTH) [108, 124], or a helper T cell response (T_H) [26, 95]. The T_C response typically is restricted by class I antigens of the major histocompatibility complex (class I MHC) [31, 110].

Table 1. Anti-idiotypic antibodies as immunologic internal images with the ability to induce protective immunity

Pathogen	Reference(s)
Escherichia coli K13	122
Experimental schistosomiasis	49
Hepatitis B	63
Human gastric cancer	53
Mycobacterium tuberculosis	95
Newcastle disease virus	125
Poliovirus type II	127
Rabies virus	94
Reovirus type 3	44, 108, 110
Sendai virus	32, 34
Streptococcus pneumoniae	26, 82
Tobacco mosaic virus	42
Trypanosoma rhodesiensis	100

Helper T cell activation by internal image anti-idiotypic antibodies is accessory cell-dependent [95] and MHC class-II-restricted [96]. Recent studies suggest that, like other T_H antigens [9], accessory cells process anti-idiotypic antibodies and present them to helper T cells in the context of MHC class II antigens [96]. Under other conditions, immunization with anti-idiotypic antibodies induces antigen-specific T_S cells [50, 83, 102, 123].

If the external antigen is the cognate ligand for a cell surface receptor, internal image anti-idiotypic antibodies may also function as anti-receptor antibodies. A large number of anti-idiotypic anti-receptor antibodies have been described, including antibodies reactive with receptors for hormones, neurotransmitters, and infectious agents (table 2). By definition such antibodies inhibit ligand-receptor binding in either a competitive or noncompetitive manner. In addition, in several systems, such antibodies have been reported to function as agonists. For example, anti-opiate receptor antibodies demonstrate agonist activity in two assays [88]. Individual antibodies reactive with the substance P receptor function as agonists for some receptors and as antagonists for others [19]. Some β-adrenergic receptor antibodies function as noncompetitive inhibitors of binding but activate adenylate cyclase [103]. Others are competitive inhibitors of binding but are antagonists of adenylate cyclase activation [54]. Some antibodies reactive with the insulin receptor [106, 111] have agonist activity in vitro where they stimulate the conversion of glucose to lipid and inhibit lipolysis in isolated adipocytes [111–113]. Also, mice developing anti-idiotypic anti-

Table 2. Internal image (anti-idiotypic) anti-receptor antibodies

Receptor class	Receptor	Reference(s)
Hormone	β-Adrenergic	54, 103
	Insulin	27, 97, 106, 111
	TSH	33, 56
	Prolactin	2
	Glucagon	97
	Vasopressin	97
Neurotransmitter	Acetylcholine	15, 131
	Substance P	19
	Dopamine	104
	Opioid	88
Microbial	Reovirus type 3	86, 89
	Murine T cell leukemia virus	3
	Polyoma virus	79
	Measles virus	66
Miscellaneous	Neutrophil chemotactic formyl peptide	75
	retinol binding protein	105, 106

insulin receptor antibodies demonstrate insulin resistance and abnormal glucose homeostasis [27]. Because anti-receptor antibodies are often easier to purify in large quantities than are natural ligands, they have proven to be useful experimental tools in a number of model systems with which to study receptor biology and the structural and functional aspects of ligand-receptor interaction.

The Reovirus Infectious Cycle

The mammalian reoviruses are ubiquitous enteric viruses, which are members of the reoviridae [58]. The reoviruses are common human pathogens; virtually 100% of adults in the general population exhibit serologic evidence of previous reovirus infection [109]. The virion consists of an icosahedral outer capsid surrounding the inner capsid and viral genome. The genome consists of 10 double-stranded RNA segments: three large segments (designated L1–3), three medium segments (designated M1–3), and four small segments (designated S1–4). Three serotypes can be distinguished on the basis of reactivity with neutralizing and anti-hemagglutination antibodies. These include strain 1 (prototype Lang), strain 2 (prototype Jones), and strain 3 (prototype Dearing). Despite overall structural similarity, the three serotypes demonstrate different routes of entry and dissemination, exhibit different patterns of tissue and cellular tropism, and mediate different diseases.

The mammalian reoviruses have been utilized to study the molecular basis of viral-host interactions because of several useful characteristics of the virus. First, with one exception, the gene segments are monocistronic. The segmented nature of the genome and the propensity of the virus to reassort upon mixed infection have greatly facilitated the mapping of phenotypic characteristics to particular gene segments and to the polypeptides encoded by them. Second, to a great extent, the pathogenesis of reovirus infection and the nature of the virus-host interaction are determined by a single viral gene segment, S1, and its product, the σ_1 outer capsid protein.

Reoviruses gain entry into the target cell by receptor-mediated endocytosis. After binding, virus-receptor complexes are taken up into phagocytic vesicles which rapidly fuse with lysosomes [115]. Uncoating occurs within the lysosome. Subviral particles directly penetrate the lysosomal membrane, enter the cytoplasm, and initiate the replicative phase of the infectious cycle [10]. Lysosomotropic agents such as NH_4Cl inhibit reovirus growth and replication [76]. Reoviruses are typically cytopathogenic. After synthesis of viral components, the virions are assembled in cytoplasmic inclusions, known as viral factories, and are released by lysis of the target cell.

The reoviruses are nonenveloped viruses. Virion budding from intracellular or plasma membranes has not been observed. However, reovirus-infected cells can serve as the targets of serotype-specific T_C [36], and a variety of viral components can be demonstrated on the surface of reovirus-infected cells. In particular, automated cytofluorometry using the neutralizing antibody, 9B.G5, confirms that the σ_1 protein is expressed on infected cells [31, 62]. The T_C response appears to be directed predominantly against the σ_1 protein as anti-σ_1 antibodies block T_C-mediated lysis [38].

Infection of mouse L fibroblasts with reovirus type 3 leads to rapid and profound inhibition of host cell DNA synthesis with relative sparing of RNA and protein synthesis [47, 107]. A decrease in the DNA synthetic rate is observed within 8–10 h after infection, prior to any visible cytopathic effects. By 24 h after infection, the DNA synthetic rate is 15–35% of mock-infected control cells. Several studies support the hypothesis that interaction of the type 3 σ_1 protein with proteins serving as the receptor for reovirus type 3 on the target cell surface (Reo3R) produces the observed metabolic effect independent of subsequent lytic infection. The binding of type 1 virus, which infects L cells equally well, has no effect on host cell DNA synthesis. Through the use of recombinant viruses, the ability to inhibit target cell growth and DNA synthesis has been genetically linked to the type 3 S1 gene segment [107]. UV-inactivated reovirus type 3, which is able to bind but has greatly reduced infectivity, retains the growth inhibiting effect [45, 107]. The binding of reovirus type 3 to B104 and R1.1 cells, which express the Reo3R but do not support productive reovirus infection, produces significant growth inhibition. Finally, anti-Reo3R antibodies and synthetic peptides corresponding to the binding regions of the σ_1 protein and 87.92.6 anti-Reo3R antibody are potent inhibitors of the growth of a variety of Reo3R-bearing cells [45, 143].

Cross-linking of receptor molecules appears to be necessary as antibody F(ab) fragments of anti-Reo3R antibodies bind to the cell surface but do not inhibit growth [45]. When monovalent F(ab) fragments are made functionally polyvalent by the addition of secondary anti-mouse Ig antibody, the growth inhibitory effect is restored. Only synthetic peptides in a form expected to produce Reo3R cross-linking are active in inhibiting growth [143]. The intracellular second messenger mediating this metabolic effect is unknown. Despite similarities between the Reo3R and the β_2-adrenergic receptor (β2AR), changes in intracellular cyclic AMP concentration do not appear to be involved.

Reoviruses typically produce acute lytic infections of target cells but under certain conditions can produce persistent productive infections both in culture [1, 8, 81] and in vivo [118]. BALB/c 3T3 fibroblasts persistently infected with reovirus appear normal at the light microscopic level but continue to release infectious virus [130]. Ultrastructural analysis demonstrates viral factories, free virus in the cytoplasm, and virus in association with lysosomes. Persistently infected cells may express viral determinants including the σ_1 protein on their surface [81, 109]. Persistently infected BALB/c 3T3 cells grow normally in serum but exhibit a decreased proliferative response to epidermal growth factor and decreased surface expression of epidermal growth factor receptor [130]. It is presently unknown which viral product mediates this effect. Also, it is unknown whether reduced expression of epidermal growth factor receptor or other cell surface receptors is similarly involved in the growth inhibition following interaction of reovirus type 3 with Reo3R during acute infection.

Reovirus type 3-specific T cell hybridomas become persistently infected after exposure to live type 3 virus [81]. When cultured in the presence of uninfected syngeneic accessory cells, the persistently infected T cell hybridomas secrete interleukin-2. Presumably, virus and/or viral components are released by these cells into the culture medium, are taken up and processed by accessory cells, and are presented to the hybridoma cells. This auto-stimulatory phenomenon is both antigen-specific and MHC class II-restricted. These findings have important implications for autoimmunity in association with viral infection.

The Reovirus σ_1 Outer Capsid Protein

The σ_1 protein is located at the 12 vertices of the icosahedral virion outer capsid and is associated with the tips of the core spikes formed by the λ_2 polypeptide. By serving as the cell attachment protein [70, 135], the σ_1 protein defines the pathways of viral entry and dissemination in the host, the cellular tropism, and the virulence of the virus [61, 120, 134, 137]. It also functions as the viral hemagglutinin [136]. Through its interaction with serotype 3-specific receptor structures on the target cell surface, the σ_1 protein mediates reovirus type 3 inhibition of target cell DNA synthesis and cell growth [107] and alteration of cellular differentiation [Cohen et al., unpublished]. Although the intact reovirus is a complex antigen, the σ_1 protein is the principal serotype-specific target antigen of both humoral [135, 136] and cellular [36] immune responses. Within the structure of the σ_1 protein, the domains which interact with somatic and immune receptors are restricted [141, 144]. These features have permitted detailed analysis of the molecular interactions between reovirus and the host organism.

Several lines of evidence demonstrate that the σ_1 protein mediates viral attachment to target cells. Serotype-specific neutralizing anti-reovirus antibodies prevent infection by blocking viral binding [70]. The antigen recognized by neutralizing antibodies maps to the S1 gene segment [135]. Neutralizing antibodies specifically immunoprecipitate the σ_1 protein [12, 121]. The σ_1 protein produced by expression of the cloned S1 gene in *E. coli* binds to L cell targets and competes with intact reovirus [80, 92]. Thus, reoviruses appear to attach to target cells via interaction of the σ_1 outer protein with cell surface structures.

The σ_1 protein also mediates reovirus binding to erythrocytes and functions as the viral hemagglutinin. Type 1 virus preferentially agglutinates human erythrocytes, while type 3 virus agglutinates bovine erythrocytes. This phenotypic characteristic maps to the S1 gene segment [136]. Hemagglutination-inhibiting antibodies specifically immunoprecipitate the σ_1 protein [12, 121]. Purified σ_1 protein is capable of agglutinating erythrocytes [80, 145]. This activity is blocked by antibodies which block the hemagglutinating activity of intact virus. Thus, the σ_1 protein mediates reovirus binding to receptor sites on both target cells and erythrocytes. As discussed below, it also plays a central role in the interaction of reovirus with immune receptors.

The S1 gene segment, which encodes the σ_1 protein, has been molecularly cloned and characterized by several laboratories [5, 13, 84]. It encompasses 1,416 nucleotides and contains two overlapping open reading frames. Both initiation sites appear to be functional. The longer open reading frame encompasses 1,365 bases, from nucleotide 13 to 1,377. The predicted protein product contains 455 amino acids with Mr = 49 kilodaltons. This value corresponds closely to the Mr of the σ_1 protein determined by sodium dodecyl sulfate/polyacrylamide gel electrophoresis (SDS/PAGE) [117].

The first 18 amino acids of σ_1 appear to comprise a signal peptide which presumably is cleaved from the processed mature protein. However, direct sequence information is unavailable because the amino-terminus is blocked. This portion of the protein contains a heptapeptide repeat pattern between amino acids 28 and 158, in which the first and fourth amino acids are hydrophobic. The remainder to the amino-terminal residues are predominantly hydrophilic. Prolines at residues 3 and 176 flank the repeat region. This sequence is typical of that of an α-helical coiled coil.

The carboxy-terminal portion of the molecule is relatively hydrophilic with clusters of hydrophobic residues. It contains 12 prolines and multiple amino acids with aromatic side chains. The predicted tertiary structure includes a mixture of short α-helical stretches, β sheets, random coils, and multiple turns. Overall, these characteristics predict a globular structure. Biochemical studies of the σ_1 protein isolated from reovirus-infected L cells and of cloned σ_1 expressed in *E. coli* suggest that in the virion the polypeptide exists as a multimer [7].

Distinct antigenic epitopes, which appear to correspond to functional domains of the σ_1 protein, have been delineated by examining the specificity pattern of serotype 3 σ_1-specific monoclonal antibodies. By determining the ability of a panel antibodies to neutralize virus and to inhibit virus-induced hemagglutination [12] and by determining the ability of antibodies to compete with one another for binding to virus [121], four groups of antibodies can be distinguished. Group I antibodies have neutralizing activity but no hemagglutination-inhibition activity. Group II antibodies inhibit hemagglutination but do not neutralize virus. Group III antibodies have both activities, and group IV have neither. Group I and II antibodies both compete with group III but not with one another. These results suggest that the neutralizing domains and hemagglutination domains are distinct functionally and topographically. Group III antibodies probably bind to an intermediate location and are able to interact with both regions. Group IV antibodies appear to interact with a distinct domain.

Studies of neutralizing antibody-resistant viral mutants have also provided information regarding the functional domains of the σ_1 protein. Variant K, derived from reovirus type 3 grown in the presence of the neutralizing antibody, 9B.G5, exhibits loss of antibody binding, altered cellular tropism, and reduced virulence [119]. Substitution of G to A at nucleotide 1,267 of the S1 gene produces a Glu to Lys change at residue 419 of the σ_1 protein [6]. This finding suggests that the residues which interact with neutralizing antibodies and with the reovirus binding site on the target cell surface are in the carboxy-terminal portion of the σ_1 protein. Studies described below confirm that this is the case.

Serotype-Specific Pattern of Cellular Tropism

The mammalian reoviruses have proven particularly useful in the study of the mechanisms determining viral tropism. The reovirus serotypes display distinct target cell specificities which reflects the high-affinity, serotype-specific interaction of the viral σ_1 protein with target cell surface receptor structures [29, 70, 87]. Serotype-specific differences in the σ_1 protein and the differential expression of serotype-specific receptor structures on potential target cells determine, in large part, the cellular tropism pattern of the virus. Within the neonatal rodent central nervous system, type 1 virus infects ependymal cells lining the ventricular system leading to a benign hydrocephalus [64, 77]. In contrast, reovirus type 3 infects neurons and glia leading to an acute panencephalitis [22, 78, 93]. The pattern of cellular tropism within the central nervous system correlates with the serotype of the S1 gene segment [137]. The use of recombinant viruses has allowed precise genetic mapping of the tropism pattern. Recombinants which contain the type 3 S1 segment on a type 1 background, designated 1HA3, display the tropism of type 3. The reciprocal recombinant displays type 1 tropism. Thus, the serotype-specific cellular tropism maps to the S1 gene segment which encodes the σ_1 outer capsid protein.

Binding studies have indicated that serotypes 1 and 3 utilize distinct receptors on most cells. Within the central nervous system, ependymal cells express receptors for reovirus type 1. Neurons and glial express receptors for serotype 3 [22, 86, 89, 129]. Mouse L fibroblasts bear distinct receptors for reovirus type 1 and 3 [29]. Intestinal epithelial cells bear receptors for reovirus type 1 but not 3 [133].

Reoviruses also exhibit a characteristic pattern of tropism for cells of the immune system. Certain murine T cell lines, including R1.1, BW5147, and EL-4, bear receptors for type 3 but not type 1 [89]. Serotype 3 but not 1 binds to murine splenic lymphocytes and human peripheral blood lymphocytes [138]. This difference in tropism maps to the S1 segment. The proportion of B cells which express binding sites for reovirus type 3 is greater than the proportion of unselected T cells [138]. Among murine spleen cells 55% of B cells but only 26% of unselected T cells bind virus. Within the T cell population, a much greater proportion of Lyt2,3(+) cells (81%) than Lyt1(+) (16%) express receptor as determined by viral binding [30] or binding of anti-Reo3R antibody [89].

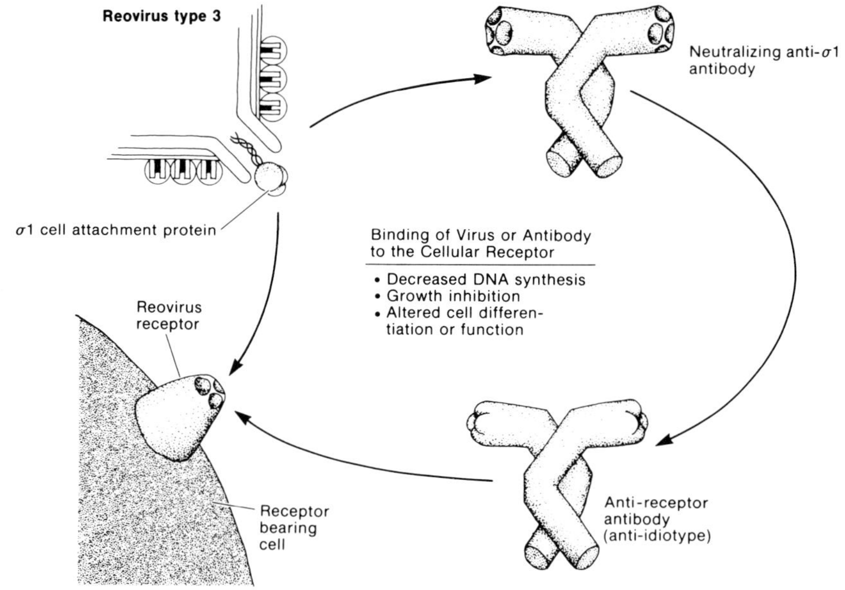

Fig. 1. Internal image anti-Reo3R antibodies. The interaction of reovirus type 3 with serotype-specific cell surface receptor structures is depicted. This interaction, which is mediated by the viral σ_1 protein, produces inhibition of target cell growth and altered cellular differentiation and function. Anti-receptor antibodies, generated as anti-idiotypes reactive with anti-σ_1 antibodies, function as functional, structural, and immunologic internal image mimics of the external antigen, the σ_1 protein.

Anti-receptor antibodies recognize the reovirus binding site expressed on neurons in primary cultures and splenic lymphocytes [8, 13, 23, 30, 86, 89], demonstrating these proteins to be antigenically related. Also, biochemical studies of the Reo3R expressed by the murine thymoma line, R1.1, and the rat neuroblastoma cell line, B104, suggest that the cell surface proteins recognized by these antibodies have similar molecular weights [16]. Thus, lymphocytes and neuronal cells express biochemically similar proteins which serve as serotype-specific reovirus binding sites (fig. 1).

Anti-Reovirus and Anti-Reovirus Receptor Antibodies

Although the reovirus is a complex antigen, the anti-reovirus immune response is directed against a small number of epitopes on a small number of proteins. As for other viruses [132, 140], the capsid proteins are the main target of immune response. Although a humoral immune response to the σ_3

and λ_2 proteins can be detected, the primary target of both the humoral [135, 136] and cell-mediated [36] immune responses to reovirus is the σ_1 outer capsid protein. The limited heterogeneity of the anti-reovirus immune response has allowed precise molecular dissection of the specificity of this response. The cellular interactions involved in the anti-reovirus immune response are summarized in figure 2.

The σ_1 protein is the dominant antigen in the humoral response to reovirus. Studies of a panel of experimentally produced mouse monoclonal anti-σ_1 antibodies have demonstrated dominant antigenic domains on the type 3 σ_1 protein [12, 121]. The neutralizing antibody, 9B.G5, is of particular interest. This antibody abrogates reovirus type 3 infectivity without affecting reovirus type 1 [12, 69, 121]. Treatment of virus particles with 9B.G antibody blocks binding to target cells [70]. Thus, it appears that the neutralizing activity of the 9B.G5 antibody results from its ability to bind to the type 3 σ_1 protein at or near the cell attachment domain and inhibit viral adsorption to target cells.

These findings suggested a potential strategy by which antibody probes for the reovirus type 3 receptor could be developed. Anti-idiotypic antibodies were isolated which react with 9B.G5 (fig. 1) in the hope of generating anti-Reo3R antibodies. Several lines of evidence demonstrate that both the xenogeneic rabbit antiserum anti-ID3 [86] and the mouse monoclonal antibody 87.92.6 [89] generated in this way are immunologic, structural, and functional mimics of the σ_1 protein and recognize a reovirus type 3 binding site important in the infectious process. Both forms of anti-Reo3R antibody have tissue and cellular binding patterns similar to that of intact virus [23, 86]. The binding parameters of anti-Reo3R antibody and intact reovirus type 3 are comparable. There are approximately 79,000 binding sites for 87.92.6 on mouse R1.1 thymoma cells with a $K_d = 9.6 \times 10^{-10}$ *M* [43], in good agreement with earlier studies of the binding of intact reovirus to these cells [29]. The binding of 87.92.6 to R1.1 and rat B104 neuroblastoma cells is blocked by reovirus type 3 [43, 60]. Anti-receptor antibodies block viral binding to neurons in culture and prevent infection [23]. Analysis of membrane extracts of R1.1 and B104 cells by SDS/PAGE and immunoblotting demonstrates that reovirus and 87.92.6 bind to proteins of similar electrophoretic mobility [16]. Immunoprecipitation studies of both cell lines using reovirus type 3 or anti-Reo3R antibodies demonstrate a single glycoprotein with Mr = 65 kilodaltons and a heterogeneous isoelectric point of 5.8–6.0. Thus, these antibodies appear to recognize cell surface structures which function as receptors for reovirus type 3.

The 87.92.6 antibody also mimics structural features of the viral σ_1 protein. The nucleic acid and deduced amino acid sequences of the type 3 σ_1 protein [5, 13, 84] and the 87.92.6 anti-Reo3R antibody [11] have been

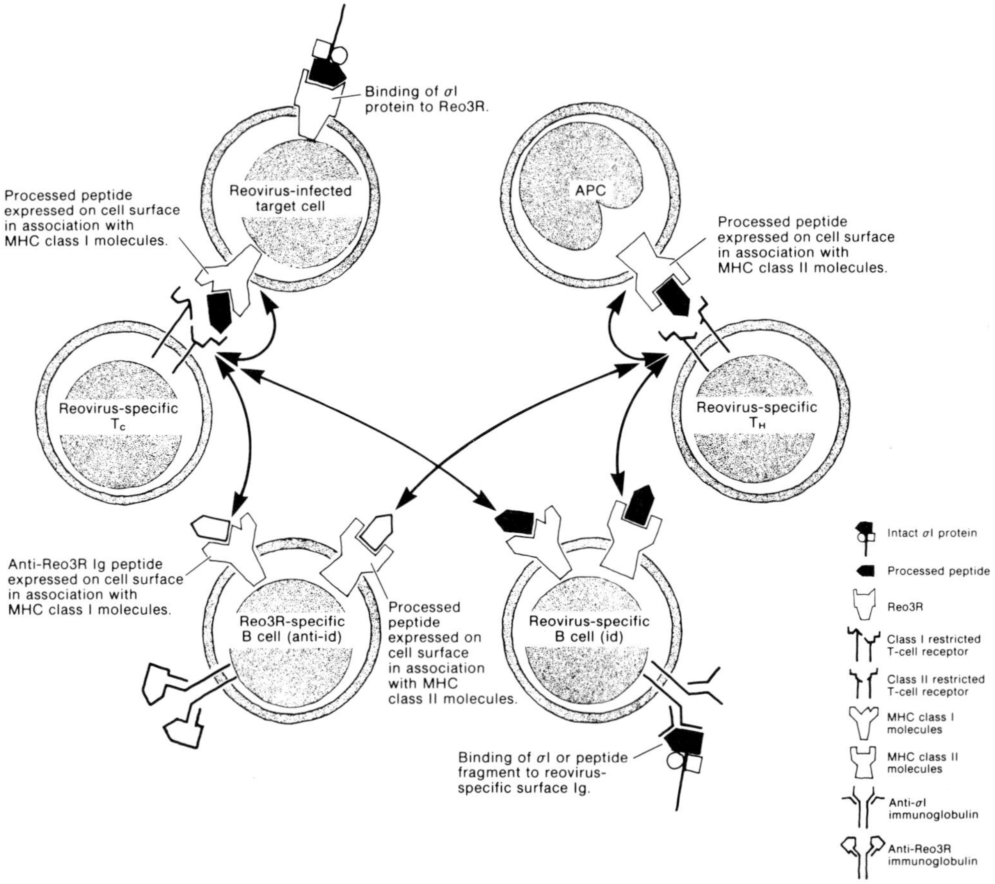

Fig. 2. The idiotypic network and cellular immune response to reovirus. Reovirus type 3-specific T_C recognize σ_1 determinants expressed on the surface of infected target cells in association with MHC class I molecules. Reovirus type 3-specific T_H cells recognize σ_1 determinants expressed on the surface of accessory cells in the context of MHC class II molecules. 87.92.6 hybridoma cells (anti-id) function as immunologic mimics of the nominal antigen. Such cells, expressing internal image antibody or processed immunoglobulin fragments in association with MHC class I and II molecules, can be recognized by reovirus type 3-specific T_C and T_H, respectively. We hypothesize that 9B.G5 cells (id), expressing neutralizing anti-σ_1 antibody, are capable of binding and internalizing the σ_1 protein via their surface immunoglobulin. After processing, peptide determinants of the σ_1 protein are expressed on the cell surface in association with MHC class I and II molecules.

determined. Substantial sequence similarity exists between a combined determinant comprised of the second complementarity determining regions (CDR II) of the heavy and light chain variable regions (V_H and V_L) and amino acids 317–332 of the type 3 σ_1 protein (fig. 3). Therefore, we postulated that these regions of sequence similarity represent the cell binding domains of the type 3 σ_1 protein and its internal image antibody, 87.92.6. Recent studies described below confirm that this is the case. Briefly, synthetic peptides corresponding to the shared amino acid sequences compete with both intact reovirus type 3 and 87.92.6 antibody for binding to the 9B.G5 neutralizing antibody and to the cell surface Reo3R [144]. These peptides also reproduce the Reo3R-mediated effects on cell growth induced by reovirus type 3 binding [143; Cohen et al., unpublished data].

Cellular Immune Response to Reovirus

The T_C response to reovirus is MHC class-I-restricted and is generally serotype-specific. However, there is some serotype cross-reactivity. Several lines of evidence suggest that the major serotype-specific target antigen is the σ_1 protein and that the major epitope recognized by T_C is the antibody neutralizing domain. The serotype-specificity is linked to the S1 gene segment [36]. Also, T_C-target cell interaction is blocked in a serotype-specific manner by anti-σ_1 antibodies [38]. Only monoclonal antibodies which recognize the neutralizing domain (A2 and G5) block T_C lysis of target cells [37]. Antibodies directed against the hemagglutinin domain (F4, F7) or other structural domains (B11, H3) do not block lysis.

The 87.92.6 antibody represents an internal image of the type 3 σ_1 domain recognized by the neutralizing antibody, 9B.G5. Interestingly, reovirus type 3-specific T_C can also lyse 87.92.6 hybridoma cells [31, 110]. This lysis is antigen-specific and MHC class-I-restricted. Between 27 and 39% of T_C clones which lyse reovirus type 3-infected P815 targets also lyse 87.92.6 hybridoma cells. Thus, the epitope shared by the σ_1 protein and the 87.92.6 antibody is a dominant epitope in the T_C response. Lysis can be blocked by preincubation of targets with 9B.G5 [31] or of effectors with 87.92.6 [110]. Thus, serotype-specific T_C lysis is blocked by anti-H2 antibodies, anti-reovirus antibodies, and anti-idiotypic anti-Reo3R antibodies. These results suggest that T_C generated after virus infection could lyse cells expressing anti-idiotypic structures.

Reovirus type 3-specific T_C which lyse 87.92.6 hybridoma cells stain uniformly by automated cytofluorometry with 87.92.6 [110]. Neither reovirus-specific T_C which do not lyse the hybridoma cells nor Sendai-virus-specific T_C stain. Thus, a proportion of type 3-specific T_C express an idiotope recognized by 87.92.6 that is shared with the 9B.G5 antibody.

However, the physiologic role of cell-mediated immunity in clearance of virus remains unclear. UV-irradiated mice are deficient in Ia-bearing adherent spleen cells and have depressed anti-reovirus type 1 T_C, DTH, and T-cell proliferative responses [72]. Nevertheless, they clear virus normally after p.o. or i.p. inoculation.

After immunization with reovirus under appropriate conditions, T cell-proliferative and DTH responses can also be demonstrated [48, 139]. Under other conditions antigen-specific suppressor cells are generated. These responses are largely MHC class II-restricted and mediated by Thy1(+) lymphocytes.

The helper T cell (T_H) and T_{DTH} responses to reovirus are generally serotype-specific and directed against antigenic determinants of the σ_1 protein, but there is some level of cross-reactivity [108, 139]. Anti-idiotypic antibody is an effective mimic of intact virus in the generation of the T_{DTH} response. Mice immunized with as little as 0.1 μg of purified 87.92.6 antibody injected in the footpads in saline in the absence of adjuvant exhibit an anti-reovirus DTH response [108]. This response is serotype-specific; no response to type 1 virus is elicited. 87.92.6 is able to prime for a response to 1HA3 virus (expressing the type 3 σ_1 on a type 1 background) but not for a response to 3HA1 (expressing the type 1 σ_1 on a type 3 background), strongly suggesting that the response is primarily directed against the σ_1 protein.

As for other antigens [25, 83], quantitative and qualitative parameters of the immune response to reovirus are determined by the dose and the route of immunization. Inoculation of adult mice with live or UV-inactivated reovirus type 1 s.c. and i.p. and live virus i.v. leads to a prominent DTH response on subsequent challenge. In contrast, immunization with UV-inactivated virus i.v. leads to serotype-specific tolerance due to the generation of Thy1(+) T_S cells [48]. Serotype-specific tolerance can also be generated by p.o. administration of UV-inactivated type 1 virus [99]. Tolerance can be adoptively transferred by Thy1(+) mesenteric lymph node cells and splenic lymphocytes. The serotype-specificity maps to the S1 gene segment, indicating that the principal target antigen is the σ_1 protein. However, only viruses with the type 1 M2 gene segment and its product, the μ_1C outer capsid protein, can generate tolerance after p.o. inoculation. This is most likely due to the resistance to digestion this protein confers. This observation illustrates how viral proteins other than the target antigen can affect the immune response to virus.

Interaction of type 3 virus with spleen cells in vitro also leads to the generation of suppressor cells [40]. Live and UV-inactivated reovirus type

3 but not serotype 1 inhibit the in vitro proliferative response of mouse spleen cells to concanavalin A. Studies using recombinant viruses confirm that this property maps to the type 3 S1 gene segment. The inhibition of the proliferative response is due to the generation of Thy1(+) suppressor T cells (T_S) cells. The generation but not the function of such cells can be inhibited in this system by the addition of anti-reovirus antibodies. As discussed above, T cells involved in the proliferative response also may express the somatic Reo3R, suggesting the possibility that the growth inhibition may be due in part to direct interaction of ligands with this receptor.

The cellular interactions involved in the anti-reovirus type 3 immune response are depicted in figure 2. The binding of reovirus to target cells is mediated by the σ_1 outer capsid protein. The σ_1 also represents the principal target antigen of the neutralizing antibody, T_H, and T_C responses to virus, although the dominant epitopes for these responses differ. Reovirus-infected target cells express σ_1 determinants on their membrane. Expression in the context of self MHC class I molecules permits recognition by reovirus type 3-specific T_C. Because of shared structural features, anti-idiotypic antibodies represent immunologic mimics of the σ_1 protein. B cells synthesizing these antibodies express these determinants either in the form of intact immunoglobulin or as processed peptide fragments in association with MHC class I. Thus, a proportion of reovirus-specific T_C are capable of lysing anti-idiotype-bearing B cells. Also, it is possible that reovirus or viral components bind to and are taken up by B cells bearing σ_1-specific antibody. Such cells might serve as targets of reovirus-specific T_C by virtue of expression of processed viral determinants on their surface.

Processed σ_1 protein is recognized by reovirus-specific T_H cells on the surface of accessory cells in the context of self MHC class II. B cells can similarly present processed peptide fragments. B cells which express anti-σ_1 antibody could induce T_H activation by virtue of their ability to bind, process, and present σ_1 determinants. Anti-idiotypic B cells could induce T_H activation by virtue of their ability to present processed internal image immunoglobulin peptide fragments. Activation of these T_H would be expected to have a positive regulatory effect on the generation of both idiotypic and anti-idiotypic antibodies.

Structural and Functional Domains Shared by the σ_1 and 87.92.6 Binding Sites

Amino acids 317–332 of the type 3 σ_1 protein exhibit striking sequence similarity to a combined determinant formed by the second complementarity determining regions of the 87.92.6 heavy and light chain variable regions

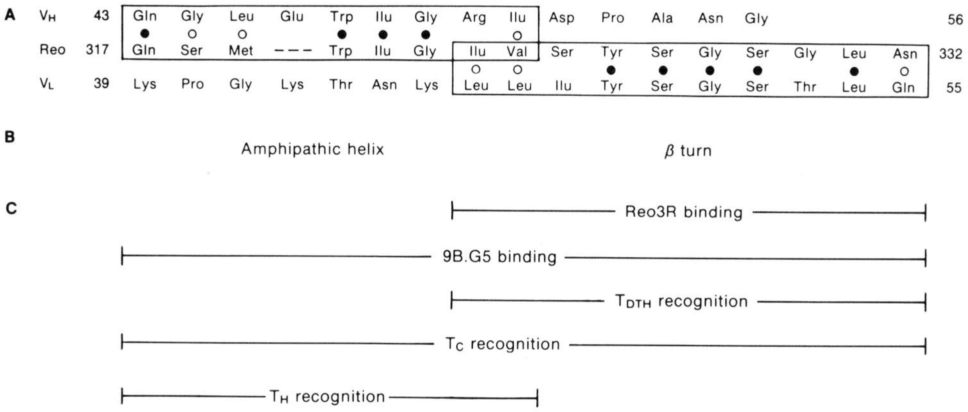

Fig. 3. Sequence similarity of the reovirus type 3 σ_1 protein and 87.92.6 antibody binding domains. *a* Comparison of the type 3 σ_1 and 87.92.6 amino acid sequences. The predicted amino acid sequence of the putative cell attachment domain of the type 3 σ_1 protein (amino acids 317–322) is presented. This sequence exhibits striking similarity to a combined determinant formed by the second complementarity-determining regions of the heavy and light chain variable domains of the anti-reovirus receptor antibody, 87.92.6 [11]. *b* The predicted tertiary structures of the V_H and V_L domains. Application of the Chou and Fasman [14] algorithm predicts that the V_H domain forms an amphipathic helix. The V_L domain appears to form a reverse β turn. *c* Functional domains of the putative type 3 σ_1 protein binding region. On the basis of studies utilizing synthetic peptides, described in the text, the domain encompassing amino acids 317–332 of the type 3 σ_1 protein can be subdivided into distinct functional domains.

[11]. As shown in figure 3a, amino acids 43–51 of the V_H CDR II are similar to amino acids 317–324 of the σ_1 protein. Amino acids 46–55 of the V_L CDR II are similar to amino acids 323–332 of the σ_1 protein. Use of synthetic peptides corresponding to these regions has permitted the mapping of functional characteristics to specific structural domains of these proteins.

Of particular interest is the sequence, Tyr-Ser-Gly-Ser, present in the putative binding regions of both the σ_1 and V_L proteins. Application of the Chou and Fasman [14] algorithm to the σ_1 and 87.92.6 sequences predicts that this region folds into a reverse turn in the two proteins (fig. 3b). This observation focused attention on this region as a potentially important sequence in the interaction of the σ_1 protein and its immunologic mimic, 87.92.6, with anti-σ_1 antibodies and with the Reo3R. The region of sequence shared by the σ_1 protein and with 87.92.6 V_H CDR II is predicted to form an amphipathic helix. This structure is a common feature of determinants recognized by helper T cells [9]. To test these hypotheses, four synthetic peptides were constructed: V_L peptide corresponds to amino acids

39–55 of 87.92.6 V_L CDR II. V_H peptide corresponds to amino acids 43–56 of 87.92.6 V_H CDR II. The V_H-V_L peptide was constructed by adding amino terminal cysteine residues to the V_H and V_L peptides allowing them to be covalently coupled. Reo peptide corresponds to amino acids 317–332 of the σ_1 protein. Unfortunately, this peptide is extremely hydrophobic making its use in anything other than solid phase assays difficult.

In competitive solid phase radioimmunoassay (RIA) employing microtiter wells coated with the 9B.G5 antibody, V_L peptide effectively and specifically inhibits the binding of radiolabelled reovirus type 3 [141, 142]. V_H-V_L peptide also is effective, but no more so on a molar basis than V_L. V_H peptide does not inhibit the interaction of reovirus type 3 with 9B.G5. Direct interaction of peptides with 9B.G5 has also been demonstrated. In solid-phase RIA employing radiolabelled 9B.G5 antibody and microtiter plates coated with peptide, specific binding of antibody to Reo, V_L, and V_H-V_L peptides but not V_H peptide can be demonstrated [141, 142]. In competitive binding studies, the V_H-V_L peptide is a more potent inhibitor than is V_L peptide in preventing 9B.G5 binding to Reo, V_L, and V_H-V_L peptides. Interestingly, V_H peptide apparently can interact with 9B.G5 in the liquid phase, as it also can specifically inhibit binding of antibody to the other peptides. These studies suggest that interaction of the σ_1 protein with the 9B.G5 antibody is mediated principally by amino acids 323–332 of σ_1, corresponding to the V_L domain of 87.92.6 but may involve the V_H domain. The interaction of 87.92.6 with 9B.G5 probably involves both the V_H and V_L domains.

Infection leads to the production of serotype-specific anti-reovirus antibodies [135]. Neutralizing anti-reovirus type 3 antibodies can also be induced by immunization with the internal image anti-idiotypic antibody, 87.92.6 [44]. Antibodies reactive with the V_L, V_H-V_L, and Reo peptides can be demonstrated after immunization with intact reovirus [144]. Conversely, immunization with V_L peptide coupled to chicken serum albumin or with Reo peptide alone leads to the production of antibodies which bind to and neutralize reovirus type 3. These antibodies also recognize the V_L, V_H-V_L, and Reo peptides in solid phase RIA. Immunization with V_H-V_L peptide, not coupled to carrier protein, leads to the production of antibodies which bind to V_H-V_L and V_L peptides but not to V_H. Immunization with V_H or V_L peptides alone does not lead to the production of anti-peptide antibodies. Taken together, these results suggest that the V_L peptide domain represents the dominant B cell epitope in vivo. The V_H peptide domain may be required to maintain the V_L domain in a particular conformation. Alternatively, it may serve an additional role in the interaction with the immune system, i.e. interaction with antigen-specific T_H cells which provide B cell help (see below).

Similar analysis of the interaction of the σ_1 protein with the Reo3R of R1.1 cells has also been carried out [141, 142]. These studies demonstrate that the V_L peptide is the most efficient inhibitor of reovirus type 3 binding to the Reo3R. V_H-V_L peptide also is effective, but no more so on a molar basis than V_L. V_H peptide does not compete with intact virus for Reo3R.

The synthetic peptides also have been utilized to analyze molecular constraints on ligand-induced Reo3R perturbation. The binding of reovirus type 3 to both B and T lymphocytes leads to capping and internalization of the Reo3R [28]. V_L peptide with an amino-terminal cysteine residue added (V_L-SH peptide) to allow peptide dimerization and Reo3R cross-linking also can down-modulate Reo3R from the target cell surface [143]. Cross-linking of Reo3R by the binding of reovirus type 3 or anti-Reo3R leads to inhibition of the growth of a number of cells which express the receptor [45, 47, 107]. In addition, Reovirus type 3 and anti-Reo3R antibodies inhibit the concanavalin A-induced lymphocyte proliferative response [87, 107]. V_L peptide dimers similarly inhibit cell proliferation [143; Cohen et al., unpublished data]. Using a panel of peptide analogs, we have begun to determine more precisely which amino acid residues and which side chains are critical for interaction of ligand with the Reo3R to produce the growth inhibitory effect [143]. V_L peptide missing the hydroxyl groups on the serine and threonine residues at positions 12 and 15 respectively demonstrates reduced ability to inhibit cell growth. Removal of the hydroxyl groups from the tyrosine and serine groups at positions 11 and 14 has little effect. Interestingly, substitution of alanine for glycine at position 13 augments the growth inhibitory action.

The interactions of 87.92.6 with 9B.G5 and Reo3R have also been studied [141, 142]. In a competitive RIA employing microtiter plates coated with 87.92.6, the ability of varying amounts of peptide to inhibit the binding of radiolabelled 9B.G5 was determined. Both V_H and V_L peptides inhibit 9B.G5 binding. However, V_H-V_L peptide is more effective. This finding indicates that both the V_H CDR II and the V_L CDR II are likely to be involved in this idiotype anti-idiotype interaction. However, when the binding of 87.92.6 to R1.1 cell surface Reo3R is studied, a different pattern is observed. While V_H-V_L peptide is more potent inhibitor of 87.92.6 binding than V_L peptide, V_H peptide does not alter 87.92.6-Reo3R interaction. Thus, both the V_L and V_H domains are involved in the 87.92.6-9B.G5 interaction. In contrast, although the V_H domain may function to maintain the necessary conformation of V_L, the latter appears to be more important in the 87.92.6-Reo3R interaction.

As described above, variant K was derived from reovirus type 3 grown in the presence of the 9B.G5 neutralizing antibody [119]. Substitution of G to A at nucleotide 1,267 of the S1 gene produces a Glu to Lys change at residue 419 of the σ_1 protein [6]. Although variant K exhibits reduced 9B.G5 antibody binding, altered cellular tropism, and reduced virulence, it competes with type 3 virus for L cell receptor sites [141]. Like type 3 virus, the binding of variant K to L cells is inhibited by V_L peptide. Thus, it appears that residue 419 of the type 3 σ_1 protein may also be involved in the binding to 9B.G5. Nevertheless, residues 317–332 appear to be more important in the interaction of the σ_1 with Reo3R.

Immunization of mice with irradiated 87.92.6 hybridoma cells leads to the production of T_C which are capable of lysing reovirus type 3-infected target cells [108]. Reovirus type 3-specific T_C are also capable of lysing targets passively coated with V_H-V_L peptide but not targets coated with either the V_H or V_L peptides alone [144]. Thus, reovirus-specific T_C appear to recognize a combined epitope corresponding to the V_H plus V_L domains in the context of MHC class I determinants.

Immunization with V_L and Reo peptides but not V_H peptides primes mice for a DTH response to intact reovirus type 3 but not type 1 [144]. The target antigen is the type 3 σ_1 protein, as demonstrated by the finding that these mice respond to the 1HA3 recombinant virus but not to 3HA1. Similarly, immunization with 1HA3 but not 3HA1 virus leads to a DTH response to V_L peptide. Thus, the V_L domain appears to be the dominant epitope involved in the DTH response to reovirus type 3.

In contrast, the V_H domain appears to be the predominant helper T cell determinant. As described above, the humoral response to the Reo peptide appears to be directed principally against the V_L domain. The V_H domain appears to be necessary for the generation of T cell help for antibody production. After immunization of mice with V_H or V_L peptides alone, lymph node cells exhibit a selective in vitro proliferative response to the immunizing peptide. However, after immunization with Reo peptide, lymph node cells proliferate in response to Reo peptide and V_H but not V_L. After immunization with 87.92.6 antibody, lymph node cells exhibit proliferative and interleukin-2 responses to intact 87.92.6 antibody and V_H peptide but not to V_L peptide. Similarly, after systemic infection with reovirus type 3, spleen cells exhibit a proliferative response to 87.92.6 antibody and V_H peptide but no response to V_L peptide. Thus, the V_H domain appears to play an important role in the T_H recognition of the type 3 σ_1 protein and of its immunologic mimic, 87.92.6.

Studies mapping the functional domains of putative binding regions of the type 3 σ_1 protein and its immunologic mimic, 87.92.6, are summarized in figure 3. These studies confirm the importance of residues 317–332 of the type 3 σ_1 protein in the interaction with immune receptors and with the somatic Reo3R (fig. 2, 3). The 87.92.6 antibody can be considered 'ligand-like', and the 9B.G5 antibody can be considered 'receptor-like'. However, there appear to be important differences between the 87.92.6 antibody and the σ_1 protein and between the 9B.G5 antibody and the Reo3R. Interaction of the σ_1 protein with the Reo3R appears to be mediated primarily by the V_L domain. In contrast, the interaction of 9B.G5 with the σ_1 protein appears to involve amino acid residue 419 of the latter and may involve the V_H domain in addition to residues 323–332. The 87.92.6–Reo3R and 9B.G5–87.92.6 interactions appear to involve both the V_H and V_L domains of 87.92.6.

Amino acids 323–332 of the σ_1 protein, the residues exhibiting the closest similarity to amino acids 46–55 of the V_L peptide, appear to comprise the domain recognized by cells mediating the DTH response and the domain most important in σ_1-Reo3R interaction. Amino acid residues 317–324, the domain corresponding to amino acids 43–51 the V_H peptide, appear to form the predominant epitope recognized by T_H cells. The binding site of the 9B.G5 antibody appears to encompass the V_L domain and possibly the V_H domain and amino acid 419. T_C appear to recognize the combined V_H plus V_L epitope. Alternatively, the V_H segment may serve to stabilize the V_L segment in the conformation necessary for interaction with the 9B.G5 antibody and the T_C antigen receptor.

The Somatic Cell Surface Receptor

Several lines of evidence suggest that the Reo3R recognized by anti-receptor antibodies and the β2AR are structurally related but probably distinct proteins. Anti-Reo3R antibodies specifically immunoprecipitate β2AR affinity purified from calf lung [17]. β-adrenergic ligands bind to immunoprecipitated Reo3R in a specific manner [17, 73]. The proteins have a similar apparent Mr = 65 kilodaltons, pl = 5.8–6.0, and tryptic digest maps. Expression of the two receptors is closely linked. Mouse R1.1 thymoma cells, hamster DDT_1 smooth muscle cells, and rat L6 myoblasts express substantial numbers of Reo3R and β2AR [Greene et al., unpublished results]. This tissue distribution of Reo3R, as defined by immunohistochemical staining of tissue sections, corresponds to that of β2AR, as defined by pharmacologic binding assays and northern blot analysis [Cohen et al., unpublished results]. In cultures of embryonic rat hypothalamic neurons, the cell populations expressing immunoreactive Reo3R and β2AR overlap closely [129]. Thus, the Reo3R and β2AR are closely related structurally and antigenically and have similar distribution patterns.

However, it appears that the virus and catecholamine-binding sites are distinct. Anti-Reo3R antibodies and β-adrenergic ligands do not compete for binding sites on either immunoprecipitated Reo3R or affinity purified

β2AR [17, 73]. The functional consequences of binding also are different. Whereas, the binding of catecholamines typically leads to the activation of adenylate cyclase and the intracellular accumulation of cyclic AMP, the binding of reovirus type 3 leads to inhibition of DNA synthesis and altered cell growth. Reovirus does not inhibit isoproterenol-induced cyclic AMP accumulation in DDT_1 cells [101].

It appears that, in addition to the β2AR, other cell surface proteins may be recognized by anti-Reo3R antibodies and may function as serotype-specific reovirus binding sites. For example, rat B104 neuroblastoma cells and mouse L fibroblasts express substantial numbers of Reo3R, as indicated by binding studies utilizing anti-Reo3R antibodies and intact reovirus type 3, but express very few β2AR [16, 29, 45, 101]. We hypothesize that these proteins are also members of the rhodopsin-like family of proteins with multiple hydrophobic transmembrane segments. Studies to identify these proteins are in progress.

Although distinct, the proteins serving as somatic Reo3R, the reovirus type 3-specific B cell receptor (typified by the 9B.G5 antibody), and MHC class I and II-restricted reovirus type 3-specific T cell antigen receptors must share certain structural features. All bind peptides derived from the type 3 σ_1 protein or its internal image mimic, the 87.92.6 antibody. Studies described above demonstrate that the immunologic and functional mimicry of the σ_1 protein by 87.92.6 results from structural mimicry at the level of primary amino acid sequence. It will be of great interest to compare the predicted amino acid sequences of the proteins which bind the σ_1 protein.

Implications for Potential Autoimmune Mechanisms

The interaction of virus with the host organism is a complex process including viral entry, dissemination, and lytic infection of target cells. In some cases, persistent productive or latent infection may be set up. A fundamental step in this process is binding to structures on host cells serving as viral receptor sites. In addition, this interrelationship involves interaction with the host immune system mediated by recognition of virus by lymphoid receptor proteins. The mammalian reoviruses represent a well-characterized model for many of these phenomena. The studies presented above have several important implications.

A variety of normal cell surface structures have been postulated to function as viral receptors (table 3). Many of these proteins are receptors for soluble mediators. Thus, interaction of virus or viral components with these structures might lead to alteration in target cell growth, differentiation, or mature function via normal or aberrant activation of existent

Table 3. Cell surface molecules proposed as virus receptors

Virus	Proposed Receptor	Reference(s)
Epstein-Barr virus	C3d receptor	41, 85
	MHC class II	98
HIV-1	CD4	20, 65
Lactic dehydrogenase virus	Ia	55
	Fc receptor	55
Rabies virus	nicotinic acetylcholine receptor	71
Reovirus type 3	β_2-adrenergic receptor	17

Table 4. Anti-receptor antibodies associated with human disease

Receptor	Disease	Reference
β_2-Adrenergic receptor	asthma, allergic rhinitis	128
C3d receptor	rheumatoid arthritis	4
FSH receptor	amenorrhea	21
Gastrin receptor	pernicious anemia	21
Insulin receptor	diabetes mellitus	39
Nicotinic acetylcholine receptor	myasthenia gravis	52
PTH receptor	secondary hyperparathyroidism	59
Transferrin receptor	iron deficiency anemia	68
TSH receptor (agonists)	Graves disease	116
(antagonists)	primary myxedema	24

second messenger mechanisms. These effects could occur independent of subsequent cytopathic infection.

Prominent inhibition of target cell growth occurs early in reovirus type 3 infection as a result of interaction of the σ_1 protein with cell surface receptor molecules related to the β2AR. Experimentally produced anti-Reo3R antibodies are similarly active. We have postulated that analogous anti-receptor antibodies generated as anti-idiotypes during the normal immune response to virus could recognize a surface structures on a variety of cells [35]. Binding of these antibodies to cell surface receptor structures could produce functional consequences, possibly at a time and anatomic location distant from the viral infection. Anti-receptor antibodies have been implicated in several human diseases (table 4). However, the origin of these antibodies remains unknown. It is of great interest that auto-antibodies reactive with a number of tissues have been demonstrated following immunization of mice with either reovirus type 1 [51, 90] or type 3 [126]. Whether such antibodies arise as anti-idiotypes remains unproven at the present time. Also, no clinicopathologic sequelae were noted in these animals. However, recent work in our laboratory demonstrates that anti-Reo3R antibodies alter oligodendrocyte differentiation in culture [Cohen et al., unpublished data] and produce primary demyelination in vivo [18]. In addition, a proportion of the cells of the immune system express the somatic reovirus receptor. The binding of reovirus or anti-Reo3R antibodies to these cells could alter immune function independent of interaction with antigen receptor.

An additional potential autoimmune mechanism is illustrated by the auto-stimulatory behavior exhibited by persistently infected T cell hybridomas. Analogous mechanisms could produce persistently infected immune cells in vivo. Accumulation of these activated cells in an inflammatory site may play a role in the production tissue damage.

Conclusions

Several characteristics of the reoviruses have facilitated the molecular analysis of virus-host interaction in this experimental system. These studies have benefited from the practical application of the idiotypic network paradigm. Conversely, studies of the mammalian reoviruses have helped elucidate the nature of the interaction of idiotype with anti-idiotype, the immune mechanisms which regulate the production of anti-idiotypic antibodies, and the functional consequences idiotypic mechanisms.

References

1 Ahmed, R.; Graham, A.F.: Persistent infections in L cells with temperature-sensitive mutants of reovirus. J. Virol. *23:* 250–262 (1977).

2 Amit, T.; Barkey, R.J.; Gavish, M.; Youdim, M.B.H.: Antiidiotypic antibodies raised against anti-prolactin (PRL) antibodies recognize the PRL receptor. Endocrinology *118:* 835–843 (1986).

3 Ardman, B.; Khiroya, R.H.; Schwartz, R.S.: Recognition of a leukemia-related antigen by an antiidiotypic antiserum to an anti-gp70 monoclonal antibody. J. exp. Med. *161:* 669–686 (1985).

4 Barel, M.; Kahan, A.; Charriaut-Marlangue, C.; Kahan, A.; Frade, R.: Autoantibodies against gp140, the Epstein-Barr virus and C3d receptor in sera from rheumatoid arthritis patients. Eur. J. Immunol. *16:* 1357–1361 (1986).

5 Bassel-Duby, R.; Jayasuriya, A.; Chatterjee, D.; Sonenberg, N.; Maizel, J.V., Jr.; Fields, B.N.: Sequence of reovirus haemagglutinin predicts a coiled-coil structure. Nature *315:* 421–423 (1985).

6 Bassel-Duby, R.; Spriggs, D.R.; Tyler, K.L.; Fields, B.N.: Identification of attenuating mutations on the reovirus type 3 S1 double-stranded RNA segment with a rapid sequencing technique. J. Virol. *60:* 64–67 (1986).

7 Bassel-Duby, R.; Nibert, M.L.; Homcy, CJ.; Fields, B.N.; Sawutz, D.G.: Evidence that the sigma 1 protein of reovirus serotype 3 is a multimer. J. Virol. *61:* 1834–1841 (1987).

8 Bell, T.M.; Ross, M.G.R.: Persistent latent infection of human embryonic cells with reovirus type 3. Nature *212:* 412–414 (1966).

9 Benjamin, D.C.; Berzofsky, J.A.; East, I.J.; Gurd, F.R.N.; Hannum, C.; Leach, S.J.; Margoliash, E.; Michael J.G.; Miller, A.; Prager, E.M.; Reichlin, M.; Sercarz, E.E.; Smith-Gill, S.J.; Todd, P.E.; Wilson, A.C.: The antigenic structure of proteins: a reappraisal. A. Rev. Immunol. *2:* 67–101 (1984).

10 Borsa, J.; Monash, B.D.; Sargent, M.D.; Copps, T.P.; Lievaart, P.A.; Szekely, J.G.: Two modes of entry of reovirus particles into cells. J. gen. Virol. *45:* 161–170 (1979).

11 Bruck, C.; Co, M.S.; Slaoui, M.; Gaulton, G.N.; Smith, T.; Fields, B.N.; Mullins, J.I.; Greene, M.I.: Nucleic acid sequence of an internal image-bearing monoclonal anti-idiotype and its comparison to the sequence of the external antigen. Proc. natn. Acad. Sci. USA *83:* 6578–6582 (1986).

12 Burstin, S.J.; Spriggs, D.R.; Fields, B.N.: Evidence for functional domains on the reovirus type 3 hemagglutinin. Virology *117:* 146–155 (1982).

13 Cashdollar, L.W.; Chmelo, R.A.; Wiener, J.R.; Joklik, W.K.: Sequences of the S1 genes of the three serotypes of reovirus. Proc. natn. Acad. Sci. USA *82:* 24–28 (1985).

14 Chou, P.Y.; Fasman, G.D.: Prediction of protein conformation. Biochemistry *13:* 222–245 (1974).

15 Cleveland, W.L.; Wasserman, N.H.; Sarangarajan, R.; Penn, A.S.; Erlanger, B.F.: Monoclonal antibodies to the acetylcholine receptor by a normally functioning auto-anti-idiotypic mechanism. Nature *305:* 56–57 (1983).

16 Co, M.S.; Gaulton, G.N.; Fields, B.N.; Greene, M.I.: Isolation and biochemical characterization of the mammalian reovirus type 3 cell-surface receptor. Proc. natn. Acad. Sci. USA *82:* 1491–1498 (1985).

17 Co, M.S.; Gaulton, G.N.; Tominaga, A.; Homcy, C.J.; Fields, B.N.; Greene, M.I.: Structural similarities between the mammalian β-adrenergic and reovirus type 3 receptors. Proc. natn. Acad. Sci. USA *82:* 5315–5318 (1985).

18 Cohen, J.A.; Sergott, R.C.; Geller, H.M.; Brown, M.J.; Greene, M.I.: Mammalian reovirus receptor expression by oligodendrocytes. Ann. N.Y. Acad. Sci. *540:* 445–448 (1988).

19 Couraud, J.-Y.; Escher, E.; Regoli, D.; Imhoff, V.; Rossignol, B.; Pradelles, P.: Anti-substance P anti idiotypic antibodies. Characterization and biological activities. J. biol. Chem. *260:* 9461–9469 (1985).

20 Dalgleish, A.G.; Beverley, P.C.L.; Clapham, P.R.; Crawford, D.H.; Greaves, M.F.; Weiss, R.A.: The CD4 (T4) antigen is an essential component of the receptor for the AIDS retrovirus. Nature *312:* 763–767 (1984).

21 De Baets, M.H.; Breda Vriesman, P.J.C. van: Autoimmunity to cell membrane receptors. Surv. Synth. Path. Res. *4:* 185–215 (1985).

22 Dichter, M.A.; Weiner, H.L.: Infection of neuronal cell cultures with reovirus mimics in vitro patterns of neurotropism. Ann. Neurol. *16:* 603–610 (1984).

23 Dichter, M.A.; Weiner, H.L.; Fields, B.N.; Mitchell, G.; Noseworthy, J.; Gaulton, G.; Greene, M.I.: Antiidiotype antibody to reovirus binds to neurons and protects from viral infection. Ann. Neurol. *19:* 555–558 (1986).

24 Drexhage, H.A.; Bottazzo, G.F.; Bitensky, L.; Chayen, J.; Doniach, D.: Thyroid growth-blocking antibodies in primary myxoedema. Nature *289:* 594–596 (1981).

25 Eichmann, K.: Idiotype suppression. I. Influence of the dose and of the effector function of anti-idiotypic antibody on the production of an idiotype. Eur. J. Immunol. *4:* 296–302 (1974).

26 Eichmann, K.; Rajewsky, K.: Induction of T and B cell immunity by anti-idiotypic antibody. Eur. J. Immunol. *5:* 661–666 (1975).

27 Elias, D.; Maron, R.; Cohen, I.R.; Shechter, Y.: Mouse antibodies to the insulin receptor developing spontaneously as anti-idiotypes. II. Effects on glucose homeostasis and the insulin receptor. J. biol. Chem. *259:* 6416–6419 (1984).

28 Epstein, R.L.; Powers, M.L.; Weiner, H.L.: Interaction of reovirus with cell surface receptors. III. Reovirus type 3 induces capping of viral receptors on murine lymphocytes. J. Immun. *127:* 1800–1803 (1981).

29 Epstein, R.L.; Powers, M.L.; Bogart, R.B.; Weiner, H.L.: Binding of ^{125}I-labelled reovirus to cell surface receptors. Virology *133:* 46–55 (1984).

30 Epstein, R.L.; Finberg, R.; Powers, M.L.; Weiner, H.L.: Interaction of reovirus with cell surface receptors. IV. The reovirus type 3 receptor is expressed predominantly on murine lyt-2,3+ and human T8+ cells. J. Immun. *133:* 1614–1617 (1984).

31 Ertl, H.C.J.; Greene, M.I.; Noseworthy, J.H.; Fields, B.N.; Nepom, J.T.; Spriggs, D.R.; Finberg, R.W.: Identification of idiotypic receptors on reovirus-specific cytolytic T cells. Proc. natn. Acad. Sci. USA *79:* 7479–7483 (1982).

32 Ertl, H.C.J.; Finberg, R.W.: Sendai virus-specific T-cell clones: induction of cytolytic T cells by an anti-idiotypic antibody directed against a helper T-cell clone. Proc. natn. Acad. Sci. USA. *81:* 2850–2854 (1984).

33 Farid, N.R.; Briones-Urbina, R.; Nazrul-Islam, M.: Biologic activity of anti-thyrotropin anti-idiotypic antibody. J. Cell Biochem. *19:* 305–313 (1982).

34 Fenner, M.; Siegmann, K.; Binz, H.: Monoclonal antibodies specific for Sendai virus. II. Production of monoclonal anti-idiotypic antibodies. Scand. J. Immunol. *24:* 341–349 (1986).

35 Fields, B.N.; Greene, M.I.: Genetic and molecular mechanisms of viral pathogenesis: Implications for prevention and treatment. Nature *300:* 19–23 (1982).

36 Finberg, R.; Weiner, H.L.; Fields, B.N.; Benacerraf, B.; Burakoff, S.J.: Generation of cytolytic T lymphocytes after reovirus infection: role of S1 gene. Proc. natn. Acad. Sci. USA *76:* 442–446 (1979).

37 Finberg, R.; Spriggs, D.R.; Fields, B.N.: Host immune response to reovirus: CTL recognize the major neutralization domain of the viral hemagglutinin. J. Immun. *129:* 2235–2238 (1982).

38 Finberg, R.; Weiner, H.L.; Burakoff; S.J.; Fields, B.N.: Type-specific reovirus antiserum blocks the cytotoxic T-cell-target cell interaction: evidence for the association of the viral hemagglutinin of a nonenveloped virus with the cell surface. Infect. Immunity *31:* 646–649 (1981).

39 Flier, J.S.; Kahn, C.R.; Jarrett, D.B.; Roth, J.: Characterization of antibodies to the insulin receptor. A cause of insulin-resistant diabetes in man. J. clin. Invest. *58:* 1442–1449 (1976).

40 Fontana, A.; Weiner, H.L.: Interaction of reovirus with cell surface receptors. II. Generation of suppressor T cells by the hemagglutinin of reovirus type 3. J. Immun. *125:* 2660–2664 (1980).

41 Frade, R.; Barel, M.; Ehlin Henriksson, B.; Klein, G.: gp140, the C3d receptor of human B lymphocytes, is also the Epstein-Barr virus receptor. Proc. natn. Acad. Sci. USA *82:* 1490–1493 (1985).

42 Francotte, M.; Urbain, J.: Induction of anti-tobacco mosaic virus antibodies in mice by antiidiotypic antibody. J. exp. Med. *160:* 1485–1494 (1984).

43 Gaulton, G.; Co, M.S.; Greene, M.I.: Anti-idiotypic antibody identifies the cellular receptor of reovirus type 3. J. Cell Biochem. *28:* 69–78 (1985).

44 Gaulton, G.N.; Sharpe, A.H.; Chang, D.W.; Fields, B.N.; Greene, M.I.: Syngeneic

monoclonal internal image anti-idiotopes as prophylactic vaccines. J. Immun. *137:* 2930–2936 (1986).
45 Gaulton, G.N.; Greene, M.I.: Inhibition of cellular DNA synthesis by reovirus occurs by a receptor-linked signalling pathway which is mimicked by anti-receptor antibody (submitted for publication).
46 Geha, R.S.: Presence of auto-anti-idiotypic antibody during the normal human immune response to tetanus toxoid antigen. J. Immun. *129:* 139–144 (1982).
47 Gomatos, P.J.; Tamm, I.: Macromolecular synthesis in reovirus-infected cells. Biochim. biophys. Acta *72:* 651–653 (1963).
48 Greene, M.I.; Weiner, H.L.: Delayed hypersensitivity in mice infected with reovirus. II. Induction of tolerance and suppressor T cells to viral specific gene products. J. Immun. *125:* 283–287 (1980).
49 Grzych, J.M.; Capron, M.; Lambert, P.H.; Dissous, C.; Torres, S.; Capron, A.: An anti-idiotype vaccine against experimental schistosomiasis. Nature *316:* 74–76 (1985).
50 Harvey, M.A.; Adorini, L.; Miller, A.; Sercarz, E.E.: Lysozyme-induced T-suppressor cells and antibodies have a predominant idiotype. Nature *281:* 594–596 (1979).
51 Haspel, M.V.; Onodera, T.; Prabhakar, B.S.; Horita, M.; Suzuki, H.; Notkins, A.L.: Virus-induced autoimmunity: monoclonal antibodies that react with endocrine tissues. Science *220:* 304–306 (1983).
52 Heinemann, S.; Bevan, S.; Kullberg, R.; Lindstrom, J.; Rice, J.: Modulation of acetylcholine receptor by antibody against the receptor. Proc. natn. Acad. Sci. USA *74:* 3090–3094 (1977).
53 Herlyn, D.; Ross, A.H.; Koprowski, H.: Anti-idiotypic antibodies bear the internal image of a human tumor antigen. Science *232:* 100–102 (1986).
54 Homcy, C.J.; Rockson, S.G.; Haber, E.: An antiidiotype antibody that recognizes the β-adrenergic receptor. J. clin. Invest. *69:* 1147–1154 (1982).
55 Inada, T.; Mims, C.A.: Ia antigens and Fc receptors of mouse peritoneal macrophages as determinants of susceptibility to lactic dehydrogenase virus. J. gen. Virol. *66:* 1469–1477 (1985).
56 Islam, M.N.; Pepper, B.M.; Briones-Urbina, R.; Farid, N.R.: Biological activity of anti-thyrotropin anti-idiotypic antibody. Eur. J. Immunol. *13:* 57–63 (1983).
57 Jerne, N.K.: Towards a network theory of the immune system. Ann. Immunol. *125C:* 373–389 (1974).
58 Joklik, W.K.: The Reoviridae (Plenum Press, New York 1983).
59 Juppner, H.; Bialasiewicz, A.A.; Hesch, R.D.: Autoantibodies to parathyroid hormone receptor. Lancet *ii:* 1222–1224 (1978).
60 Kauffman, R.S.; Noseworthy, J.H.; Nepom, J.T.; Finberg, R.; Fields, B.N.; Greene, M.I.: Cell receptors for the mammalian reovirus. II. Monoclonal anti-idiotypic antibody blocks viral binding to cells. J. Immun. *131:* 2539–2541 (1983).
61 Kauffman, R.S.; Wolf, J.L.; Finberg, R.; Trier, J.S.; Fields, B.N.: The σ_1 protein determines the extent of spread of reovirus from the gastrointestinal tract of mice. Virology *124:* 403–410 (1983).
62 Kauffman, R.S.; Lee, S.; Finberg, R.: Cytolytic T-cell mediated lysis of reovirus-infected cells: requirements for infectious virus, viral particles, and viral proteins in infected target cells. Virology *131:* 265–273 (1983).
63 Kennedy, R.C.; Dreesman, G.R.: Enhancement of the immune response to hepatitis B surface antigen. In vivo administration of antiidiotype induces anti-HBs that express a similar idiotype. J. exp. Med. *159:* 655–665 (1984).
64 Kilham, L.; Margolis, G.: Hydrocephalus in hamsters, ferrets, rats, and mice following inoculations with reovirus type 1. I. Virologic studies. Lab. Invest. *21:* 183–188 (1969).

65 Klatzmann, D.; Champagne, E.; Chamaret, S.; Gruest, J.; Guetard, D.; Herscend, T.; Gluckman, J.C.; Montagnier, L.: T-lymphocyte T4 molecule behaves as the receptor for human retrovirus LAV. Nature *312:* 767–768 (1984).
66 Krah, D.L.; Choppin, P.W.: Mice immunized with measles virus develop antibodies to a cell surface receptor for binding virus. J. Virol. *62:* 1565–1572 (1988).
67 Kunkel, H.G.; Mannik, M.; Williams, R.C.: Individual antigenic specificities of isolated antibodies. Science. *140:* 1218–1219 (1963).
68 Larrick, J.W.; Hyman, E.S.: Acquired iron-deficiency caused by antibody against the transferrin receptor. New Engl. J. Med. *311:* 214–218 (1984).
69 Lee, P.W.K.; Hayes, E.C.; Joklik, W.K.: Characterization of anti-reovirus immunoglobulins secreted by cloned hybridoma cell lines. Virology *108:* 134–146 (1981).
70 Lee, P.W.K.; Hayes, E.C.; Joklik, W.K.: Protein σ_1 is the reovirus cell attachment protein. Virology *108:* 156–163 (1981).
71 Lentz, T.L.; Burrage, T.G.; Smith, A.L.; Crick, J.; Tignor, G.H.: Is the acetylcholine receptor a rabies virus receptor? Science *215:* 182–184 (1982).
72 Letvin, N.L.; Kauffman, R.S.; Finberg, R.: T lymphocyte immunity to reovirus: cellular requirements for generation and role in clearance of primary infections. J. Immun. *127:* 2334–2339 (1981).
73 Liu, J.; Co, M.S.; Greene, M.I.: Reovirus type 3 and ^{125}I-iodocyanopindolol bind to distinct domains on the beta-adrenergic receptor. Immunol. Res. (in press).
74 Ludwig, D.S.; Finkelstein, R.A.; Karu, A.E.; Dallas, W.S.; Ashby, E.R.; Skoolnik, G.K.: Anti-idiotypic antibodies as probes of protein active sites: application to cholera toxin subunit B. Proc. natn. Acad. Sci. USA *84:* 3673–3677 (1987).
75 Marasco, W.A.; Becker, E.L.: Anti-idiotype as antibody against the formyl peptide chemotaxis receptor of the neutrophil. J. Immun. *128:* 963–968 (1982).
76 Maratos-Flier, E.; Goodman, M.J.; Murray, A.H.; Kahn, C.R.: Ammonium inhibits processing and cytotoxicity of reovirus, a nonenveloped virus. J. clin. Invest. *78:* 1003–1007 (1986).
77 Margolis, G.; Kilham, L.: Hydrocephalus in hamsters, ferrets, rats, and mice following inoculations with reovirus type 1. II. Pathologic studies. Lab. Invest. *21:* 189–198 (1969).
78 Margolis, G.; Kilham, L.; Gonatas, N.K.: Reovirus type III encephalitis: observations of virus-cell interactions in neural tissues. I. Light microscopy studies. Lab. Invest. *24:* 91–100 (1971).
79 Marriott, S.J.; Roeder, D.J.; Consigli, R.A.: Anti-idiotypic antibodies to a polyomavirus monoclonal antibody recognize cell surface components of mouse kidney cells and prevent polyomavirus infection. J. Virol. *61:* 2747–2753 (1987).
80 Masri, S.A.; Nagata, L.; Mah, D.C.W.; Lee, P.W.K.: Functional expression in *Escherichia coli* of cloned reovirus S1 gene encoding the viral cell attachment protein 1. Virology *149:* 83–90 (1986).
81 Matsuzaki, N.; Hinshaw, V.S.; Fields B.N.; Greene, M.I.: Cell receptors for the mammalian reovirus: reovirus-specific T-cell hybridomas can become persistently infected and undergo autoimmune stimulation. J. Virol. *60:* 259–266 (1986).
82 McNamara, M.K.; Ward, R.E.; Kohler, H.: Monoclonal idiotope vaccine against *Streptococcus pneumoniae* infection. Science *226:* 1325–1326 (1984).
83 Monroe, J.G.; Gurish, M.; Dambrauskas, J.; Slaoui, M.; Lowy, A.; Greene, M.I.: Genetic and biological characterization of a T suppressor cell induced by anti-idiotypic antibody. J. Immun. *135:* 1589–1597 (1985).
84 Nagata, L.; Masri, S.A.; Mah, D.C.W.; Lee, P.W.K.: Molecular cloning and sequencing of the reovirus (serotype 3) S1 gene which encodes the viral cell attachment protein 1. Nucl. Acids Res. *12:* 8699–8710 (1984).

85 Nemerow, G.R.; Wolfert, R.; McNaughton, M.E.; Cooper, N.R.: Identification and characterization of the Epstein-Barr virus receptor on human B lymphocytes and its relationship to the C3d complement receptor (CR2). J. Virol. *55:* 347–351 (1985).
86 Nepom, J.T.; Weiner, H.L.; Dichter, M.A.; Tardieu, M.; Spriggs, D.R.; Gramm, C.F.; Powers, M.L.; Fields, B.N.; Greene, M.I.: Identification of a hemagglutinin-specific idiotype associated with reovirus recognition shared by lymphoid and neural cells. J. exp. Med. *155:* 155–167 (1982).
87 Nepom, J.T.; Tardieu, M.; Epstein, R.L.; Noseworthy, J.H.; Weiner, H.L.; Gentsch, J.; Fields, B.N.; Greene, M.I.: Virus-binding receptors: similarities to immune receptors as determined by anti-idiotypic antibodies. Surv. immunol. Res. *1:* 255–261 (1982).
88 Ng, D.S.S.; Isom, G.E.: Anti-morphine anti-idiotypic antibodies. Opiate receptor binding and isolated tissue responses. Biochem. Pharm. *34:* 2853–2858 (1985).
89 Noseworthy, J.H.; Fields, B.N.; Dichter, M.A.; Sobotka, C.; Pizer, E.; Perry, L.L.; Nepom, J.T.; Greene, M.I.: Cell receptors for the mammalian reovirus. I. Syngeneic monoclonal anti-idiotypic antibody identifies a cell surface receptor for reovirus. J. Immunol. *131:* 2533–2538 (1983).
90 Onodera, T.; Rayh, U.R.; Melez, K.A.; Suzuki, H.; Toniolo, A.; Notkins, A.L.: Virus-induced diabetes mellitus: autoimmunity and polyendocrine disease prevented by immunosuppression. Nature *297:* 66–68 (1982).
91 Oudin, Y.; Michael M.: Une nouvelle forme d'allotypie des globulins du sérum de lapin apparement liée à la fonction et à la spécificité antecorps. C.R. Acad Sci. *257:* 805–808 (1963).
92 Pelletier, J.; Nicholson, R.; Bassel-Duby, R.; Fields, B.N.; Sonenberg, N.: Expression of reovirus type 3 (Dearing) σ_1 and σ_s polypeptides in *Escherichia coli.* J. gen. Virol. *68:* 135–145 (1987).
93 Raine, C.S.; Fields, B.N.: Reovirus type III encephalitis – a virologic and ultrastructural study. J. Neuropath. exp. Neurol. *32:* 19–33 (1973).
94 Reagan, K.J.; Wunner, W.H.; Wiktor, T.J.; Koprowski, H.: Anti-idiotypic antibodies induce neutralizing antibodies to rabies virus glycoprotein. J. Virol. *48:* 660–666 (1983).
95 Rees, A.D.M.; Praputpittaya, K.; Scoging, A.; Dobson, N.; Ivanyi, J.; Young, D.; Lamb, J.R.: T-cell activation by anti-idiotypic antibody: evidence for the internal image. Immunology *60:* 389–393 (1987).
96 Rees, A.D.M.; Scoging, A.; Dobson, N.; Praputpittaya, K.; Young, D.; Ivanyi, J.; Lamb, J.R.: T cell activation by anti-idiotypic antibody: mechanism of interaction with antigen-reactive T cells. Eur. J. Immunol. *17:* 197–201 (1987).
97 Reilly, T.M.; Root, R.T.: Production of idiotypic and anti-idiotypic antibodies by Balb/c mice in response to immunizations with glucagon, vasopressin, or insulin: supporting evidence for the network concept. J. Immun. *137:* 597–602 (1986).
98 Reisert, P.S.; Spiro, R.C.; Townsend, P.L.; Stanford, S.A.; Sairenji, T.; Humphreys, R.E.: Functional association of class II antigens with cell surface binding of Epstein-Barr virus. J. Immun. *134:* 3776–3779 (1985).
99 Rubin, D.; Weiner, H.L.; Fields, B.N.; Greene, M.I.: Immunologic tolerance after oral administration of reovirus: requirement for two viral gene products for tolerance induction. J. Immun. *127:* 1697–1701 (1981).
100 Sacks, D.L.; Esser, K.M.; Sher, A.: Immunization of mice against African trypanosomiasis using anti-idiotypic antibodies. J. exp. Med. *155:* 1108–1119 (1982).
101 Sawutz, D.G.; Bassel-Duby, R.; Homcy, C.J.: High affinity binding of reovirus type 3 to cells that lack beta-adrenergic receptor activity. Life Sci. *40:* 399–406 (1987).
102 Saxon, A.; Barnett, E.: Human auto-antiidiotypes regulating T cell-mediated reactivity to tetanus toxoid. J. clin. Invest. *73:* 342–348 (1984).

103 Schreiber, A.B.; Couraud, P.O.; Andre, C.; Vray, B.; Strosberg, A.D.: Anti-alprenolol anti-idiotypic antibodies bind to β-adrenergic receptors and modulate catecholamine-sensitive adenylate cyclase. Proc. natn. Acad. Sci. USA *77:* 7385–7389 (1980).

104 Schreiber, M.; Fogelfeld, L.; Souroujon, M.C.; Kohen, F.; Fuchs, S.: Antibodies to spiroperidol and their anti-idiotypes as probes for studying dopamine receptors. Life Sci. *33:* 1519–1526 (1983).

105 Sege, K.; Peterson, P.A.: Anti-idiotypic antibodies against anti-vitamin A transporting protein react with prealbumin. Nature *271:* 167–168 (1978).

106 Sege, K.; Peterson, P.A.: Use of anti-idiotypic antibodies as cell-surface receptor probes. Proc. natn. Acad. Sci. USA *75:* 2443–2447 (1978).

107 Sharpe, A.H.; Fields, B.N.: Reovirus inhibition of cellular DNA synthesis: role of the S1 gene. J. Virol. *38:* 389–392 (1981).

108 Sharpe, A.H.; Gaulton, G.N.; McDade, K.K.; Fields, B.N.; Greene, M.I.: Syngeneic monoclonal antiidiotype can induce cellular immunity to reovirus. J. exp. Med. *160:* 1195–1205 (1984).

109 Sharpe, A.H.; Fields, B.N.: Pathogenesis of viral infections. Basic concepts derived from the reovirus model. New Engl. J. Med. *312:* 486–497 (1985).

110 Sharpe, A.H.; Gaulton, G.N.; Ertl, H.C.J.; Finberg, R.W.; McDade, K.K.; Fields, B.N.; Greene, M.I.: Cell receptors for the mammalian reovirus. IV. Reovirus-specific cytolytic T cell lines that have idiotypic receptors recognize anti-idiotypic B cell hybridomas. J. Immun. *134:* 2702–2706 (1985).

111 Shechter, Y.; Maron, R.; Elias, D.; Cohen, I.R.: Autoantibodies to insulin receptor spontaneously develop as anti-idiotypes in mice immunized with insulin. Science *216:* 542–545 (1982).

112 Shechter, Y.; Elias, D.; Maron, R.; Cohen, I.R.: Mice immunized to insulin develop antibody to the insulin receptor. J. Cell Biochem. *21:* 179–185 (1983).

113 Shechter, Y.; Elias, D.; Maron, R.; Cohen, I.R.: Mouse antibodies to the insulin receptor developing spontaneously as anti-idiotypes. I. Characterization of the antibodies. J. biol. Chem. *259:* 6411–6415 (1984).

114 Shoelson, S.E.; Marshall, S.; Horikoshi, H.; Kolterman, O.G.; Rubenstein, A.H.; Olefsky, J.M.: Antiinsulin receptor antibodies in an insulin-dependent diabetic may arise as autoantiidiotypes. J. clin. Endocr. Metab. *63:* 56–61 (1986).

115 Silverstein, S.C.; Dales, S.: The penetration of reovirus RNA and initiation of its genetic function in L-strain fibroblasts. J. Cell Biol. *36:* 197–230 (1968).

116 Smith, B.R.; Hall, R.: Thyroid-stimulating immunoglobulins in Graves' disease. Lancet *ii:* 427–431 (1974).

117 Smith, R.E.; Zweerink, H.J.; Joklik, W.K.: Polypeptide components of virions, top components and cores of reovirus type 3. Virology *39:* 791–810 (1969).

118 Spandidos, D.A.; Graham, A.F.: Generation of defective virus after infection of newborn rats with reovirus. J. Virol. *20:* 234–247 (1976).

119 Spriggs, D.R.; Fields, B.N.: Attenuated reovirus type 3 strains generated by selection of haemagglutinin antigenic variants. Nature *297:* 68–70 (1982).

120 Spriggs, D.R.; Bronson, R.T.; Fields, B.N.: Hemagglutinin variants of reovirus type 3 have altered central nervous system tropism. Science *220:* 505–507 (1983).

121 Spriggs, D.R.; Kaye, K.; Fields, B.N.: Topological analysis of the reovirus type 3 hemagglutinin. Virology *127:* 220–224 (1983).

122 Stein, K.E.; Soderstrom, T.: Neonatal administration of idiotype or antiidiotype primes for protection against *Escherichia coli* K13 infection in mice. J. exp. Med. *160:* 1001–1011 (1984).

123 Sy, M.-S; Bach, B.A.; Dohi, Y.; Nisonoff, A.; Benacerraf, B.; Greene, M.I.: Antigen- and receptor-driven regulatory mechanisms. I. Induction of suppressor T cells with anti-idiotypic antibodies. J. exp. Med. *150:* 1216–1228 (1979).

124 Sy, M.-S; Brown, A.R.; Benacerraf, B.; Greene, M.I.: Antigen- and receptor-driven regulatory mechanisms. III. Induction of delayed-type hypersensitivity to azobenzenearsonate with anti-cross-reactive idiotypic antibodies. J. exp. Med. *151:* 896–909 (1980).

125 Tanaka, M.; Sasaki, N.; Seto, A.: Induction of antibodies against Newcastle disease virus with syngeneic anti-idiotypic antibodies in mice. Microbiol. Immunol. *30:* 323–331 (1986).

126 Tardieu, M.; Powers, M.L.; Hafler, D.A.; Hauser, S.L.; Weiner, H.L.: Autoimmunity following viral infection: demonstration of monoclonal antibodies normal tissue following infection of mice with reovirus and demonstration of shared antigenicity between virus and lymphocytes. Eur. J. Immunol. *14:* 561–565 (1984).

127 UytdeHaag, F.G.C.M.; Osterhaus, A.D.M.E.: Induction of neutralizing antibody in mice against poliovirus type II with monoclonal anti-idiotypic antibody. J. Immun. *134:* 1225–1229 (1985).

128 Venter, J.C.; Fraser, C.M.; Harrison, L.C.: Autoantibodies to β2-adrenergic receptors: a possible cause of adrenergic hyporesponsiveness in allergic rhinitis and asthma. Science *207:* 1361–1363 (1980).

129 Ventimiglia, R.; Greene, M.I.; Geller, H.M.: Localization of beta adrenergic receptors on differentiated cells of the central nervous system in culture. Proc. natn. Acad. Sci. USA *84:* 5073–5077 (1987).

130 Verdin, E.M.; Maratos-Flier, E.; Carpentier, J.-L.; Kahn, C.R.: Persistent infection with a nontransforming RNA virus leads to impaired growth factor receptors and response. J. cell. Physiol. *128:* 457–465 (1986).

131 Wasserman, N.H.; Penn, A.S.; Freimuth, P.I.; Treptow, N.; Wentzel, S.; Cleveland, W.L.; Erlanger, B.F.: Anti-idiotypic route to anti-acetylcholine receptor antibodies and experimental myasthenia gravis. Proc. natn. Acad. Sci. USA *79:* 4810–4814 (1982).

132 Webster, R.G.; Laver, W.G.: Preparation and properties of antibody directed specifically against the neuraminidase of influenza virus. J. Immun. *99:* 49–55 (1967).

133 Weiner, D.B.; Girard, K.; Williams, W.; McPhillips, T.; Rubin, D.H.: Reovirus type 1 and type 3 differ in their binding to isolated epithelial cells. Microb. Path. (in press).

134 Weiner, H.L.; Drayna, D.; Averill, D.R.; Fields, B.N.: Molecular basis of reovirus virulence: role of the S1 gene. Proc. natn. Acad. Sci. USA *74:* 5744–5748 (1977).

135 Weiner, H.L.; Fields, B.N.: Neutralization of reovirus: the gene responsible for the neutralization antigen. J. exp. Med. *146:* 1305–1310 (1977).

136 Weiner, H.L.; Ramig, R.F.; Mustoe, T.A.; Fields, B.N.: Identification of the gene coding for the hemagglutinin of reovirus. Virology *86:* 581–584 (1978).

137 Weiner, H.L.; Powers, M.L.; Fields, B.N.: Absolute linkage of virulence and central nervous system cell tropism of reoviruses to viral hemagglutinin. J. infect. Dis. *141:* 609–616 (1980).

138 Weiner, H.L.; Ault, K.A.; Fields, B.N.: Interaction of reovirus with cell surface receptors. I. Murine and human lymphocytes have a receptor for the hemagglutinin of reovirus type 3. J. Immun. *124:* 2143–2148 (1980).

139 Weiner, H.L.; Greene, M.I.; Fields, B.N.: Delayed hypersensitivity in mice infected with reovirus. I. Identification of host and viral gene products responsible for the immune response. J. Immun. *125:* 278–282 (1980).

140 Willcox, N.; Mautner, V.: Antigenic determinants of adenovirus capsids. I. Measurement of antibody cross-reactivity. J. Immun. *116:* 19–24 (1976).

141 Williams, W.V.; Guy, H.R.; Rubin, D.H.; Robey, F.; Myers, J.N.; Kieber-Emmons, T.; Weiner, D.B.; Greene, M.I.: Sequence of the cell-attachment sites of reovirus type 3 and its internal image and modeling of their three-dimensional structures. Proc. natn. Acad. Sci. USA *85:* 6488–6492 (1988).
142 Williams, W.V.; Guy, H.R.; Weiner, D.; Rubin, D.; Greene, M.I.: Structure of the neutralizing epitope of the reovirus type 3 hemagglutinin. Vaccines 88 (Cold Spring Harbor Press, New York, 1988).
143 Williams, W.V.; Moss, D.A.; Cohen, J.A.; Myers, J.N.; Weiner, D.B.; Greene, M.I.: Antibody domains with biological activity (submitted for publication).
144 Williams, W.V.; London, S.L.; Rubin, D.H.; Wadsworth, S.; Weiner, D.B.; Berzofsky, J.; Greene, M.I.: Immune response to a molecularly defined internal image idiotype (submitted for publication).
145 Yeung, M.C.; Gill, M.J.; Alibhai, S.S.; Shahrabadi, M.S.; Lee, P.W.K.: Purification and characterization of the reovirus cell attachment protein σ_1. Virology *156:* 377–385 (1987).

Jeffrey A. Cohen, MD, Department of Neurology, Hospital of the University of Pennsylvania, 3400 Spruce Street, Philadelphia, PA 19104 (USA)

Sercarz E (ed): Antigenic Determinants and Immune Regulation. Chem Immunol.
Basel, Karger, 1989, vol 46, pp 157–168

Suppression of the Response to Murine Alloantigens: Four-Cell-Type Clusters, Function-Flipping and Idiosyncratic Responses

N.A. Mitchison

Imperial Cancer Research Fund Tumour Immunology Unit, University College London, Department of Biology, Medawar Building, London, England

Antigen-specific immunosuppression, the subject of this article, gets reviewed fairly frequently [3, 7, 8] and the author either singly or jointly has done so on several recent occasions [2, 16, 18, 20, 23]. This article aims to avoid repetition, and certainly does not aspire to collect together all the available facts. Its purpose is rather to expose a few new ideas that have emerged out of recent work on murine alloantigens, and accordingly it is arranged into two main sections: an introductory outline, to provide a background against which these ideas can be evaluated, and then a section that develops three of them more fully.

Background: An Outline of Suppression

We start with a beginner's list of the principles of suppression.

(1) Examples of suppression keep cropping up. They can be recognised as such by means of cell-mixing experiments, in which suppressor cells impair the activity of helper cells. Sometimes the cell-mixing is done in vitro, which has the advantage that the cells that participate can be examined in detail more easily. At others it is done in vivo, where the suppressive effect is often more reliable, but the choice of method seems to be mostly a matter of taste. Sometimes investigators put the cart before the horse, and conclude in favour of suppression merely from the fact that anti-CD8 or anti-H-2E or anti-HLA-DQ treatment enhances a response, or because hybrids of high × low responders give a low response.

(2) Suppression does not crop up at random. Confronting the immune system with a large dose of antigen, preferably given intravenously, readily induces suppression. So does chronic exposure to antigen given even in quite small amounts, particularly when the response is anyway marginal. Any response to chronic immunisation that rises and then declines must

arouse a strong suspicion of suppression, a topic that we return to below. The genetics of the host is also important. Immune suppression genes (Is genes) have been identified that regulate a variety of responses; many of them are normal class II MHC genes that also serve in other responses as Ir genes, but evidence is growing of a bias towards Is function on the part of certain genes, notably H-2E in mouse and HLA-DQ in man [23].

(3) Partitioning of the suppressor cell population reveals certain generalities. A typical suppressor population consists of suppressor-inducer cells bearing the CD4 marker mixed with suppressor-effector cells bearing CD8; the latter act on CD4 helper cell targets. All are T cells, and so in mice bear the Thyl marker. Thus the starter kit for pathway analysis comprises anti-CD4, CD8, and Thyl monoclonal antibodies, all of which are now available in the form of highly cytotoxic IgM antibodies, made in rat versus mouse. But many other reagents are now entering use, particularly for splitting the CD4 and CD8 compartments, including monoclonal antibodies to CD45R (successively in rat, man, and mouse), P80 (in man), *Vicia lobosa* lectin (in mouse), and a variety of other less well characterised markers [16, 20].

(4) A problem then arises: some of these characteristics such as restriction define lineages, while others such as the CD45R phenotype define maturation or 'activation' states. In order to reconcile the two, it has been suggested that a particular restriction element may in the course of evolution come to associate with particular environmental antigens, so that T cells restricted in that way may mature preferentially [20]; but this idea lacks supporting evidence. None of the markers that split the CD4 or CD8 compartments unequivocally identifies a suppressor lineage; the strongest claims for lineage have been made on behalf of p80, but it is very difficult to satisfy oneself in this respect for markers known only on human lymphocytes.

(5) So at this point we are still in some confusion, with biases towards suppressor activity evident within subdivisions of the main CD4 T cell compartment, suggesting that it can be subdivided; but like Poland these subdivisions have no natural frontiers. It is in this connection that the issue of connectivity arises.

By the time of the last International Congress of Immunology it had become clear that T cells as a whole lock tightly into the network of B cell idiotypes [18]. This was evident in the powerful influence that immunoglobulin V regions exert on the T cell repertoire: for instance in the fine structure of allogeneic responses [28], and also in the substantial impact on T cells of anti-IgM treatment [9]. But this influence seemed to be particularly strong for suppressor activities: for instance, cell-mixing experiments would sometimes (but not always [6]) work only when the suppressor and target cells came from Ig-VH-matched hosts. We coined the term 'epirestriction' to denote this phenomenon where a gene restricts a cell-cell interaction (i.e. the two participating cells have to come from donors that have the same allele of the gene), but does so via the network so that the gene itself need not be expressed within either of the two cells [18]. The term does not seem to have caught on, but it still provides a useful way of summarising this situation. Epirestriction seemed also to apply to the I-J phenomenon as then understood: it seems particularly relevant that an H-2E transgene can alter the I-J phenotype [5].

Since that time progress continues in exploring the network. Immunoglobulin transgenes provide a powerful new tool for investigating epirestriction, and the CD5 B cell (or Lyl B cell as it is sometimes still called in mice) has been discovered to occupy a central position in the control of idiotype [10, 11, 25]. We eagerly await application of these concepts to the analysis of suppression.

So, in summary, connectivity adds to our constellation of biases, but once again we are left without anything to discriminate sharply between suppressor and other regulatory T cells.

(6) At this point in the argument a choice opens up. One could go on to construct a model of suppression based simply on the biases in markers, restriction, and connectivity as outlined above, to which might be added the distribution of different lymphokine-secretion profiles (the Thyl/Th2 classification and its ramifications [22]). This route would leave us without any cell-type or molecular mechanisms unique for suppression. We might postulate, for instance, some sort of lethargic cytolytic T cell, that kills its target helper T cell via an idiotypic interaction, or perhaps a greedy lymphokine consumer. There are plenty of possibilites, and little to decide between them. They have in common the concept of suppressor activity as a composite property, as distinct from something fundamentally unique.

Alternatively one could continue to search for a unique cell that operates a unique molecular mechanism. Such a cell might operate a new set of variable genes encoding a new type of receptor, as has been suggested [13]. This would reflect a more hopeful view, but one which has little to show for two decades of effort. The main achievement in that direction has been to identify a group of suppressor factors, soluble proteins that are released by suppressor T cells and that seem able to mediate their activity. None of these factors have been fully characterised; and none of the molecular biology that one might hope for has emerged, such as RNA processing to yield soluble T cell receptor, or class II MHC molecules in soluble form. But as a perceptive review puts it, this work on factors cannot simply be avoided [26]. My own view is that receptors and MHC molecules may well be cleaved off cell membranes more or less at random, and that they might then have some physiological function although that would be hard to demonstrate; but at the end of the day, none of that would make much difference to our ideas about the fundamental mechanism of suppression (or indeed of other immunoregulatory functions, such as epitope-linkage) unless the products of hitherto unidentified genes should be involved.

(7) The evolutionary significance of suppression is another subject of debate. At one end of the spectrum suppression can be regarded as a fundamental homeostatic mechanism, generally required for control of the immune response. At the other, it can be dismissed as a set of laboratory artefacts, of little relevance to normal operation of the immune system. We hold a view somewhere in between, that suppression has evolved to meet certain requirements imposed mainly by chronic infectious disease, and that these vary from one species to another in relation to disease burden, length of life, and other factors. One key factor in this evolution may be the need to keep part of the immune system free to deal with fresh challenges, even when confronted with large amounts of antigen from an ongoing infection, as Benjamin suggests. Another, arguably more important, factor is the need to control infection-related hypersensitivity [17]. Our view finds support in the apparent flip of suppressor function that has occurred from the HLA-DQ/H-2A to the HLA-DR/H-2E gene during the evolution of mice, as well as in the frequency with which wild mice lose H-2E expression, and it makes testable predictions about HLA-DQ gene frequencies in relation to endemic disease. But much further work is needed to test these ideas.

New Ideas: (1) Four-Cell-Type Clusters

The concepts of suppressor-epitopes and of preferential restriction of suppressor-inducer cells (by HLA-DQ or H-2E) pose an important problem: how is it possible for a suppressor T cell that recognises one epitope (presented on one MHC molecule) to inactivate a helper T cell that recognises another epitope (presented on another MHC molecule [27, 29]? In other words, how can epitope-linkage operate between suppression and help? And in particular, how can this take place if the T cells involved are linked together by an idiotype-anti-idiotype chain, as the evidence for connectivity cited above indicates? At one time these problems could perhaps be solved by postulating that mouse T cells can express (1) class II MHC molecules, and (2) more than one TcR per cell [1]; but that time has surely passed.

Clustering provides a reasonable solution to this problem. Three-cell-clusters consist of an interdigitating dendritic cell (an antigen-presenting cell), with helper T cells and cytolytic T cell precursors bound to it. They

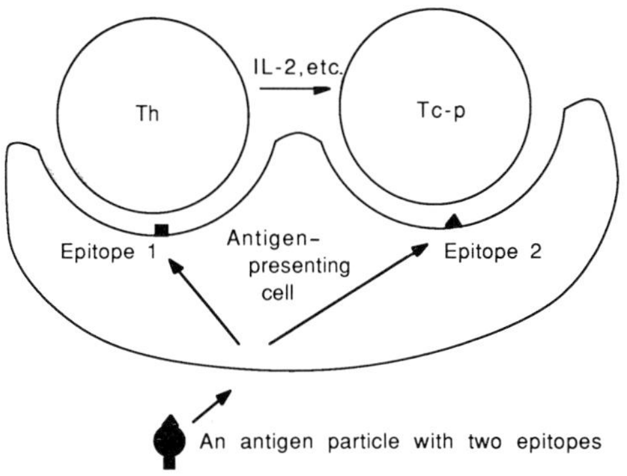

Fig. 1. Two epitopes on a single antigenic particle enter an antigen-presenting cell, presumably an interdigitating dendritic cell, where they are cleaved apart and then presented (on appropriate MHC molecules, not shown) to a helper T cell and a cytolytic T cell precursor. Lymphokines can then act at ultrashort range. This mechanism operates epitope linkage, but only under conditions where the number of antigenic particles per presenting cell are small [19]. The two types of T cell need not be cognate [19].

have not been demonstrated directly (this would not be an easy task under normal physiological conditions, although who knows what the confocal microscope may reveal), but their existence can be inferred from indirect evidence [19]. A cluster enables short-range lymphokines (IL-2, plus presumably IL-4, IL-6, and perhaps others as well) to diffuse from the regulatory cell to the effector-precursor, and thus mediate linkage between epitopes that form part of a single antigenic structure, as illustrated in figure 1. Interdigitating dendritic cells have the right combination of qualities to perform this task, for they (a) process antigen to major histocompatibility complex (MHC)-associative peptides, rather than retain it conformationally intact, (b) retain antigen for short periods (unlike B cells, T cells do not hypermutate and so do not need time to mature), and (c) are spaced well apart from one another, thus ensuring epitope linkage. Very probably the overall architecture of lymphoid tissue, with its division into T and B areas, depends on these differences between interdigitating and follicular dendritic cells; the latter have the opposite combination of qualities, fitting them well for antigen-presentation to B cells [2].

Clustering has opened a whole new area of cell biology. Two variant cells have just been discovered that provide valuable clues. One of these is the $CD2^-$, presumed $\gamma\delta$-receptor-bearing, T cell of the sheep; this cell does not enter into cluster formation with interdigitating-type dendritic cells [15]. The other is the HLA^- 'bare lymphocyte' identified as a cause of congenital immunodeficiency. Following the normal two-cell-type cluster formation of B cells with T cells, this type of B cell does not subsequently decluster in the absence of antigen [4] in the normal way. It will be appreciated that declustering has to take place smoothly, as a 'productive' cluster, i.e. one in which the right T cell clusters with the right B cell in the presence of the right antigen must occur very much less frequently than a non-productive one (just as foreplay in mammalian species other than man does not usually lead to consummation). At any rate, from these two observations a scheme of normal clustering and declustering can be constructed. Clustering commences with the binding of CD2 (on the T cell) to LFA-3 (on the antigen-presenting cell, whether B cell or interdigitating dendritic cell). Other interactions then take place, principally binding of LFA-1 to ICAM, and of TcR in combination with CD4 or CD8 to class II MHC molecules. In the presence of the appropriate antigen, activation of the T cell then takes place, whereas in its absence (the usual case) declustering follows as a result of signals transmitted presumably via the TcR.

Both CD2 and the TcR-T3 complex have been identified as signal transducers. In that process the importance of conformational change may in the past have been overestimated, in comparison with the effect of perturbation of mixed populations of transmembrane molecules. For instance, an equilibrium state of phosphorylation established in a mixture of phosphokinases and phosphatases might be perturbed by capping either enzyme; note that capping of CD2 and of CD3 at the cell interface is a characteristic feature of clustering.

On this basis we can formulate ideas about four-cell-type clusters that would solve much of the problem of suppression posed above: figure 2 illustrates one such proposal. Note that two helper T cells are involved, one of which (on the right in fig. 2) is a conventional helper cell, a Th2 cell in Mosmann's nomenclature [22], whose business it would normally be to go on and help a B cell to respond; this cell recognises H-2A molecules presenting a helper epitope. The other cell (the suppressor-inducer cell on the left) acts as a suppressor-inducer by releasing lymphokines; this cell recognises H-2E molecules presenting a suppressor epitope. The lymphokines thus released stimulate at ultrashort range the suppressor-effector cell, which then functions as an indolent cytolytic T cell and kills the conventional helper via an idiotype-anti-idiotype connection.

No doubt this proposal is open to criticism. For instance, a problem would arise if cloned suppressor cells should still display H-2E restriction, as my colleague Dr. N. Nanda believes she has discovered. And the proposal makes little distinction between Tsi and Th within the CD4 T cell set, a difference which we have previously emphasised in the foregoing account. The real purpose of presenting this proposal is to illustrate the

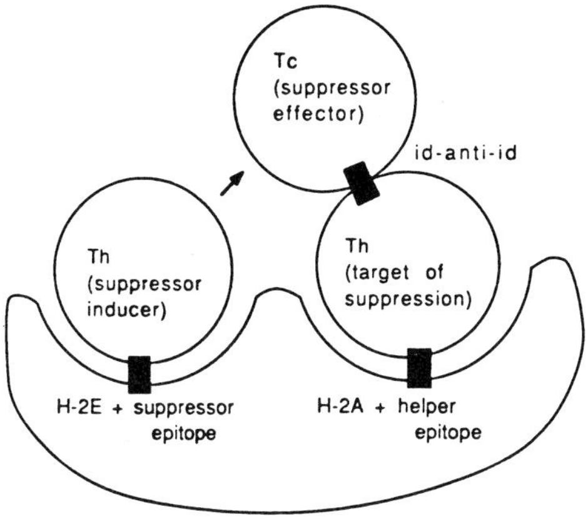

Fig. 2. A hypothetical four-cell-type cluster that would (1) mediate epitope linkage between suppressor and helper epitopes, recognised respectively by suppressor-induced and helper T cells by the same mechanism as was illustrated in figure 1, (2) avoid postulating expression of class II MHC molecules on T cells, and (3) satisfy the requirement for idiotype-anti-idiotype connection between the suppressor-effector and target (helper) cell.

new direction that these multiple clusters give to our thinking about suppressor pathways. The crucial point is that epitope linkage can still be preserved without direct adhesion of regulatory to effector cell. Once that point is accepted, numerous possibilities come to mind that can be tested only by further experiment.

New Ideas: (2) Flipping of Suppressor Function and the Mysteries of A^b

This discussion revolves around the immunological behaviour of the C57BL mouse strain, and its substrains B6 and B10. So peculiar are these mice, in any number of ways, that geneticists have long wondered whether they should really be regarded as mice at all. From these peculiarities has sprung much of the genetics of suppression, and their cornering of the market is reinforced by the fact that the most valuable recombinant strains (2R, 4R, 5R) derive from a cross between B10 and B10.A. All this is evident in our recent survey of H-2 class II immune suppression genes [23].

The immunogentics in question can be summarised as follows. Firstly, these mice have the H-2^b haplotype, within which A^b functions as a conventional Ir gene: that is to say it can bind and present to helper T cells some but not all epitopes. Secondly, these mice can perform either as high or as low responders for another reason, to do with suppression when the

MHC class II genes behave as Is genes. As high responders they do so because their other class II gene E^b is not expressed; this enables them to avoid the suppression that this gene tends to mediate when it is expressed. As low responders they perform in this way because A^b can behave in an anomalous way, through itself mediating suppression. We need to examine in some detail the evidence for this latter contention.

Before doing so, one point needs to be clarified: How different are Ir and Is functions? In the light of our introductory outline of suppression, it seems likely that class II MHC molecules perform their helper and suppressor function in fundamentally the same way, by providing a target for the receptors of CD4 T cells to recognise (in other words, by restricting the activity of these cells). But the secondary consequences of that initial step seem to be quite different, for while some activated CD4 T cells serve as suppressor-inducers, others go on to serve as classical helper T cells. In this sense we can distinguish between Ir and Is functions, while bearing in mind the way in which the two are similar.

Our evidence of Is functioning of the A^b gene emerged from a study of the antibody response to F liver protein in Fl hybrids of CBA and AKXL recombinant inbred strains [24]. In this panel all mice did make some response, as expected since they had been selected for presence of the appropriate F allele and all had at least one dose of the A^k gene, the only known Ir gene for this response. However within the observed range hybrids having the A^b gene made a low response. On its own this does not establish the A^b gene as mediating Is function and a full analysis of these genetics and the cellular responses that they mediate is still underway; but much that is already known about the immunogenetics of this particular anti-F response points in that direction [24].

Our next example of A^b seemingly functioning as an Is gene comes from a study of the response to 'pure' Thyl antigen. Fl hybrids between A strain mice and various B10 congenic strains that differ at H-2, including the recombinants 2R, 4R and 5R mentioned above, were immunised with congenic thymocytes of A.Thyl.1 origin. Here low responsiveness again segregated with the presence of A^b derived from the B10-type parent. This response is discussed in greater detail in the section below, and has not yet been published in detail.

Two swallows do not make a summer, and we certainly need to know more about other alleles at A which occur in E^- haplotypes. Nevertheless these two examples take us to a point from which we can begin to generalise. It looks as though an MHC class II molecule could perform suppressor functions in three distinct but not exclusive ways: (1) as a result of reduced expression, (2) by preferential binding to an auxiliary molecule, or (3) as a result of repertoire selection. Option (1), reduced expression, looks particularly likely in man, where HLA-DQ in contrast to HLA-DR combine a normally low level of expression with expression on a smaller range of cell types, and slower γ-interferon induction kinetics. Option (2), in the form of the CD45R molecule participating in lymphocyte activation by the TcR/MHC complex, is favoured by one active research group, but their experimental evidence for direct binding is not yet compelling [21]. Option (3), repertoire selection, provides a straighforward explanation of the anomalous behaviour of A^b as outlined above. Perhaps we are witnessing the counterpart for suppression of function flipping as it has been observed previously for help: throughout a range of haplotypes the E gene restricts the helper response to a particular epitope, and then when this gene is not expressed (E^- haplotypes) restriction flips to the A gene [12].

Where do mice stand in relation to option (1) above, reduced expression of their suppression-mediating E gene? In most haplotypes, including $H\text{-}2^k$ where E has been identified as mediating suppression, expression appears not to be reduced. Furthermore upon induction, E has been reported to respond with the same kinetics as A [30]. Nevertheless I doubt if this issue has been entirely resolved.

New Ideas: (3) Idiosyncratic Responses May Be Useful Probes of Suppression

Responses that vary greatly from one individual to another within an inbred strain are anathema to most biologists. That is why immunologists tend to pool individual sera or spleens before starting an experiment. Recent experience in immunising mice with 'pure' Thyl antigen, as outlined above, suggests that by doing so something of value may be missed.

Briefly, these Thyl congenic mice respond to numerous repeated weekly injection of Thyl antigen idiosyncratically. Some individuals make progressively higher levels of antibody, as is nearly always the case when mice are immunised with 'impure' Thyl (i.e. non-congenic Thyl antigen, such as AKR → CBA). Other individuals make some antibody early on but this later drops off while yet others hardly get started at all. Both those latter types of individual, as it turns out in cell transfer experiments, appear to have developed active suppression specific for the 'pure' antigen. The tendency of mice to respond in this way seems to be highly sensitive to immunogenetic control.

It begins to look as though suppression-inducing regimes divide into two main categories. One involves delivering a single sledgehammer blow of antigen, preferably intravenously. For allo-immunisation, typical examples would be induction of suppression by 10^8 lymphocytes allogeneic for minor histocompatibility antigens, given intraveneously [6], or induction of suppression by 3 mg of allo-F protein [14]. Typically, all individuals respond and immunogenetics have little impact. The other involves continuous sprinkling with antigen, as in the example mentioned above. Into this category also fall most or all of the instances of suppression induced by protein administered as adjuvant [24], and probably also suppression of transplantation antigens occurring in neonatal chimeras and chronic graft-versus-host disease. The significant point, but one for which we have at present only these hints of evidence, is that continuous sprinkling, by inducing an idiosyncratic response, may pick up delicate effects that the sledgehammer misses.

Summary

Specific immune suppression develops under certain well-defined conditions of exposure to antigen, where it is evident as a diminution of the immune response due to the activity of antigen-specific suppressor cells, usually T cells. Although subject to intensive study over the last two decades, interest in suppression has declined recently because of failure to make progress in defining molecular mechanisms or the precise cells involved. This review outlines present information, and then goes on to present three new ideas that emerge from study of murine alloantigens: (1) how the formation of four-cell-type clusters might mediate suppression; (2) a classification of means whereby class II MHC molecules may mediate suppression that includes a suggestion to account for the anomalous behaviour of H-2A^b; and (3) the value of idiosyncratic responses as probes of suppressor mechanisms. It does not provide an exhaustive coverage review of the literature, but recommends certain other reviews that do so.

References

1 Baxevanis, C.N.; Ishii, N.; Nagy, Z.A.; Klein, J.: H-2-controlled suppression of T cell response to lactate dehydrogenase B. Characterisation of the lactate dehydrogenase B suppressor pathway. J. exp. Med. *156:* 822–833 (1982).

2 Dexter, M.; Marvel, J.; Merkenschlager, M.; Mitchison, N.A.; Oliveira, D.B.G.; O'Malley, C.; Smith, L.; Terry, L.; Timms, E.: Progress in T cell biology. Immunol. Lett. *16:* 171–178 (1987).

3 Dorf, M.E.; Benacerraf, B.: Suppressor cells and immunoregulation. A. Rev. Immunol. *2:* 127–158 (1984).

4 Fischer, A.: Personal communication.

5 Flood, P.M.; Benoist, C.; Mathis, D.; Murphy, D.B.: Altered I-J phenotype in Eα transgenic mice. Proc. natn. Acad. Sci. USA *83:* 8308–8312 (1986).

6 Gascoigne, N.; Crispe, N.: Suppression of the cytotoxic T-cell responses to minor alloantigens in vivo. Linked recognition by suppressor T cells. Eur. J. Immunol. *14:* 210–215 (1984).
7 Germain, R.N.; Benacerraf, B.: A single major pathway of T-lymphocyte interactions in antigen-specific immune suppression. Scand. J. Immunol. *13:* 1–10 (1981).
8 Green, D.R.; Flood, P.M.; Gershon, R.K.: Immunoregulatory T-cell pathways. A. Rev. Immunol. *1:* 439–463 (1983).
9 Hayglass, K.T.; Benacerraf, B.; Sy, M.S.: T cell development in B cell-deficient mice. V. Stopping anti-μ treatment results in Igh-restricted expansion of the T suppressor cell repertoire concomitant with the development of normal immunoglobulin levels. J. exp. Med. *164:* 36–49 (1986).
10 Herzenberg, L.A.; Stall, A.M.; Lalor, P.A.; Sidman, C.; Moore, W.A.; Parks, D.R.; Herzenberg, L.A.: The Ly-l B-cell lineage. Immunol. Rev. *93:* 81–102 (1986).
11 Herzenberg, L.A.; Stall, A.M.; Braun J.; Weaver, D.; Baltimore, D.; Herzenberg, L.A.; Grosschedl, R.: Depletion of the predominant B-cell population in immunoglobulin Mμ heavy-chain transgenic mice. Nature *329:* 71–3 (1987).
12 Ishii, N.; Baxevanis, C.N.; Nagy, Z.A.; Klein, J.: Selection of H-2 molecules for the context of antigen recognition by T lymphocytes. Immunogenetics *14:* 283–292 (1981).
13 Janeway, C.: Do suppressor T cells exist? A reply. Scand. J. Immunol *27:* 621–623.
14 Lukic, M.L.; Mitchison, N.A.: Self- and allo-specific suppressor T-cells evoked by intravenous injection of F protein. Eur. J. Immunol *14:* 766–768 (1984).
15 MacKay, C.R.; Hein, W.R.; Brown, M.H.; Matzinger, P.: Unusual expression of CD2 in sheep: implications for T cell interactions. Eur. J. Immunol. *18:* 1681–1688.
16 Marvel, J.; Mitchison, N.A.; Oliveira, D.B.G.; O'Malley, C.: The split within the CD4 (helper) T-cell subset, and its implications for immunopathology. Mem. Inst. Oswaldo. Cruz. *82:* 260–273 (1987).
17 Mitchison, N.A.; Oliveira, D.B.G.: Chronic infection as a major force in the evolution of the suppressor T cell system. Parasitol. Today *2:* 312–313 (1986).
18 Mitchison, N.A.; Oliveira, D.B.G.: Epirestriction and a specialised subset of T helper cells are key factors in the regulation of T suppressor cells; in Cinader, Richard, Miller, Progress in immunology, vol. VI, pp. 326–334 (Academic Press, New York 1986).
19 Mitchison, N.A.; O'Malley, C: Three cell type clusters of T-cells with antigen-presenting cells best explain the epitope linkage and non-cognate requirements of the in vivo cytolytic response. Eur. J. Immunol. *17:* 579–583 (1987).
20 Mitchison, N.A.: Suppressor activity as a composite property. Scand. J. Immunol. (in press).
21 Morimoto, C.; Letvin, N.L.; Rudd, C.E.; Hagan, M.; Takeuchi, T.; Schlossman, S.F.: The role of the 2H4 molecule in the generation of suppressor function in Con A-activated T cells. J. Immun. *137:* 3247–3253 (1986).
22 Mosmann, T.R.; Cherwinski, H.; Bond, M.W.; Giedlin, M.A.: Coffman, R.L.: Two types of murine helper T cell clone. I. Definition according to profiles of lymphokine activities and secreted proteins. J. Immun. *136:* 2348–2537 (1986).
23 Oliveira, D.B.G.; Mitchison, N.A.: Immune suppression genes. Clin. exp. Immunol. (in press).
24 Oliveira, D.B.G.; Nardi, N.: Immune suppression genes control the anti-F antigen response in Fl hybrids and recombinant inbred sets of mice. Immunogenetics *26:* 359–365 (1987).
25 Rajewsky, K.: Evolutionary and somatic selection of the antibody repertoire in the mouse. Science *238:* 1088 (1987).
26 Schwartz, R.H.: Immune response (Ir) genes of the mouse histocompatibility complex. Adv. Immunol. *38:* 31–201 (1986).

27 Servis, C.; Seckler, R.; Nagy, Z.A.; Klein, J.: Two adjacent epitopes on a synthetic dodecapeptide induce lactate dehydrogenase B-specific helper and suppressor T cells. Proc. R. Soc. B *228:* 461–471 (1986).
28 Sherman, L.A.: The origin of strain-specific differences in the specificity repertoires of murine cytolytic T lymphocytes. J. Immun. *136:* 3977–3980 (1986).
29 Wicker, L.S.; Katz, M.; Sercarz, E.E.; Miller, A.: Immunodominant protein epitopes. I. Induction of suppression to hen egg white lysozyme is obliterated by removal of the first three N-terminal amino acids. Eur. J. Immunol. *14:* 442–447 (1984).
30 Witmer-Pack, M.D.; Valinsky, J. Olivier, W.; Steinman, R.M: Quantitation of surface antigen on cultured mouse epidermal Langerhans' cells: rapid and selective increase in the level of surface MHC products. J. invest. Derm. *90:* 387–394 (1988).

N.A. Mitchison, Imperial Cancer Research Fund Tumour Immunology Unit,
University College London, Department of Biology, Medawar Building,
Gower Street, London WC1E 6BT (England)

Sercarz E (ed): Antigenic Determinants and Immune Regulation. Chem Immunol. Basel, Karger, 1989, vol 46, pp 169–185

The Architectonics of Immune Dominance: The Aleatory Effects of Molecular Position on the Choice of Antigenic Determinants

Eli E. Sercarz[1]

Department of Microbiology, University of California, Los Angeles, Calif., USA

There is a common conception among immunologists that the specificity repertoire expressed by lymphocytes in response to antigenic determinants is controlled directly by the available repertoires of T and B cells and their affinities for ligand. This genetically deterministic view is modified to be sure by the vagaries of major histocompatibility complex (MHC) presentation of the antigen and by such modifications as mutations in antigen-driven B cells. But these amendments simply are restatements of the view that what comes out at the response end is related generally to *genomic* restrictions of the organism. Of course, it is a tautology that the organism must be capable of assembling an immune response of the quality that is eventually produced. But this view of the immune response neglects the large body of experimentation which shows that almost invariably the immune system does not play its whole repertoire when asked to give a concert.

I would like to defend an alternative view of the functioning of the system in which the designation of an antigenic determinant as dominant is an accident of molecular architecture, i.e. of the position of the determinant within the structure of the molecule. Its relationship to other determinants, the existence of strategic amino acids of importance for processing, and the hierarchy of preferential sites on the antigen for binding to MHC molecules, will each play a role in the choice of the piece(s) that will be played at the concert.

Immunodominance Is a Universal Attribute of Immune Responses

It is a reproducible fact of life of the immune system that at every point dominance effects can be perceived. That is to say, a limitation is

[1] I would like to acknowledge my first encounter with 'aleatory' as a term [66]. The work in our laboratory was supported in part by NIH grants AI-11183 and CA-24442.

observed in the expressed repertoire, although the particular subpopulation of cells is capable of response to a broader range of determinants. This is quite evident in the predominant idiotypy of most responses to antigen: single idiotopes seem to be positively selected to the exclusion of others. Again, in the responses of cytolytic, helper and suppressor T cells, there are dominant determinants that influence the complementary T cells and expand them preferentially. Likewise, the primary response to lysozyme at the B cell level is surprisingly restricted to epitopes at the amino terminus of the molecule: if the 3 amino-terminal residues are cleaved, about 50% of first-degree response antibodies bind poorly or not at all to hen egg-white lysozyme (HEL) [1]. These and other instances are summarized in table 1 and will be expanded on later. In such cases, there is no genetically limited repertoire or genetically determined lack of specific binding to MHC molecules: rather, a combination of seemingly fortuitous events conspire to direct the response in a favored direction. This recurring theme of dominance is a clue to the economy of the immune system, which we have discussed elsewhere [2]. Suffice it to say here that it must be considered wasteful to pursue a large variety of parallel responses. Surely, from the point of view of regulation, cogent control can best be exerted when there are a minimal number of responses: e.g. with thousands of idiotypic interactions having to be independently regulated, the chances for error or evasion would be enormous [3]. Therefore, one implication of this view is that dominance is so widespread because it is necessary for efficient and regulated activity of the immune system for there to be a small number of choices.

Table 1. Pervasiveness of immune dominance in different lymphocyte subpopulations

Antigen presentation (helper T cells): only certain antigenic determinants are used in a particular mouse strain despite the existence of a broader repertoire directed against others
Antigen presentation (suppressor T cells): T suppressor cells show very restricted specificity and use a different set of antigenic determinants
Idiotypic systems: predominant idiotopes characterize many antibody responses, and these B cell idiotopes are also predominant in the suppressive circuitry
Restriction element preference (MHC class II): when a peptide containing two determinants restricted by different MHC molecules is injected, usually all clones in a given line are reactive to a single, but not necessarily the same, determinant
Restriction element preference (MHC class I): in many cases, clones restricted to a single class I element will dominate
B cells (epitope dominance): the primary antibody response seems to be directed toward a limited portion of the molecule
B cells (clonal dominance): the isoelectric focusing spectrum becomes very limited in the hyperimmune response to a determinant

Antigens as Determinant Mosaics, Addressing Different Functions

Crucial in achieving this focus is a coordinated approach to dealing with the highly complex determinant mosaics found on the average protein molecule. Even on molecules as small as the lysozymes (molecular weight = 14.3 kilodaltons), many mouse strains are able to perceive a continuum of three-dimensional, discontinuous B cell determinants (BD) [4], from 4–8 helper-T-cell-inducing determinants (HD) and a small number of suppressor-T-cell-inducing determinants (SD). In two antigen systems that we have studied extensively, HEL [5] and *Escherichia coli* beta-galactosidase (GZ) [6], the HD and SD are unique and nonoverlapping. The BD characteristics of native HEL are entirely different from those HD on reduced HEL or its peptides that associate with the MHC [7]. These determinants can be considered as initiating the immune response and getting the immune machine going in first gear. Modulating forces, shifting the response into a higher gear, may be provided by other antigen-specific cells but, probably, most regularly by elements of the immune network, acting at the T or B cell level. Of course, as Gershon was wont to emphasize [8], the eventual modulation of the response has to be a braking force that brings the system back to equilibrium.

The balance between positive and negative regulation is manifest in the overall response to a multideterminant antigen. What will become evident after a discussion of HD hierarchies is that T cells directed to the dominant determinant can be either susceptible or resistant to suppression. Since the outcome of a battle for HD dominance itself is inherently unpredictable, whether there is a response or not to the whole antigen, will be equally unpredictable, at least from 'first principles'.

Presentation by the MHC and an Appropriate T Cell Repertoire – The Constituents of the Genetic Determinist View

A typical model of antigen handling pictures the native antigen binding to a structure such as the immunoglobulin receptor, being endocytosed and then fragmented randomly into peptides about 10–20 amino acids in length. These fragments then compete for binding onto the appropriate class II molecule at its peptide-binding site, are reexpressed on the surface of the cell where ambient T cells bind to sufficient ligand complexes and then are activated by signals released from the antigen-presenting cells. In this model, any peptide fragment derived from the native molecule that bears an agretope complementary to the ligand-binding site on a class II molecule will be involved in T cell activation: the variables to consider are the affinity of the various peptides for the class II site and the existence of T cells of the necessary specificity.

Let us treat the T cell repertoire problem first. Our early evidence [9–11] showed that although the number of determinant areas on lysozyme which were used by H-2^b mice was limited, within these stretches of roughly 15 amino acids, there were a multiplicity of 'epitopes', as defined in Heber-Katz et al.'s [12] strict sense of being the amino acids making contact with the T cell receptor 'paratope'. This conclusion was confirmed in many laboratories working with a large number of small protein antigens [13–16]. The corollary view is that once an agretope (the site of antigen recognition by class II) exists there should be no trouble in finding a suitable repertoire of T cells. For minimal determinants, there might be a more restricted repertoire: for example, in the response to myelin basic protein in the B10.PL mouse, the 1–9 peptide seems to be dominant, and it is recognized in conjunction with the A^u molecule [17]. When the T cell receptor repertoire was examined, a surprising restriction was found, with only two different V beta genes and two different V alpha genes being used to constitute these receptors [18, 19]. The puzzle which still has not been solved in this case concerns whether the small, amino-terminal peptide truly bears a single, rather than multiple epitopes, or whether it is a situation in which dominant T cells bearing the particular $\alpha\beta$ gene receptors are expressed while the subdominant T cells lie dormant. In any event, there is no a priori reason to believe that even a platonically ideal, single T cell epitope would have to be recognized by a single V gene constellation.

With respect to the affinity of an agretope for the complementary binding site (or 'desetope') on class II, it is difficult to dispute the supposition that this affinity has to be reasonably high to permit interaction. A direct test of binding efficiency and dominance was made in recent studies by Sette et al. [20], where a large variety of determinants restricted to a particular class II molecule were compared in binding inhibition experiments. It was demonstrated that in each case where there was a strong interaction between peptide and MHC molecule, the peptide contained a determinant which activated T cells in that strain. However, where the interaction with the MHC molecule was less affine, the proportion of peptides that actually served as T-cell-activating determinants was much lower. The reverse is not necessarily true: several cases are known where adequately strong binding to MHC does not insure the *dominance* of that determinant [21], and therefore the expression of T cells directed against it when the whole antigen is provided. One of these cases involves the E^k restriction element and the use of lysozyme peptide 81–96 as a binding inhibitor of the response of a T cell hybridoma specific for the E^k-restricted pigeon cytochrome c peptide 81–104. Although the HEL peptide is an excellent (4+) inhibitor in the scheme of Buus et al. [22], when HEL is used itself as immunogen, T cells specific for this peptide never arise although they are readily induced by the peptide itself. In such cases it is apparent that this peptide is very low on a hierarchy of availability from the native, tightly folded molecule.

The conclusion seems inescapable from both lines of evidence that the T cell repertoire rarely is the limiting factor when a strain seems to be unresponsive to a particular peptide. Nevertheless, it appears to be that during the induction of thymic tolerance, reactivities against certain antigenic molecules (for example, self-MHC and Mls) are obliterated [23–25]. Considering the large array of T cells that recognize different epitopes on a single determinant peptide on a foreign peptide and, further, factoring in the variation among the epitopes recognized on the restricting MHC molecule (the 'histotopes'), it is surprising that *all* of the T cells potentially reactive with that peptide could have been tolerized by a fortuitous cross-reactivity with a self-determinant in the context of self-MHC, unless the determinant falls into the class of 'super determinants' [26].

These host factors we have mentioned are a major component of those sine qua non ingredients that affect T cell determinant recognition *at the site* where the ternary complex of T cell receptor, MHC and antigen meet. These factors are listed in table 2. Another feature of recognition which some have considered as required, or at least highly favored, is a special secondary structure of the antigenic ligand that fits into the MHC cleft, e.g. an amphipathic alpha-helix. In this connection, it is interesting that, even among the small number of MHC haplotypes we have studied in detail, almost every portion of the HEL molecule, despite considerable variability in secondary structure along the molecule, is used by one of them. We conclude that no single secondary peptide structure characterizes a successful determinant in all haplotypes. From the point of view of the species, it is likely that different MHCs would have evolved sites of the greatest possible diversity for antigen binding. This fits the evidence of Malcolm Gefter, Howard Grey and their colleagues demonstrating that peptides binding to different isotypic restriction elements, e.g. A^d and E^d, have characteristic motifs with distinctive patterns of hydrophobicity and charge [27, 28].

Table 2. Factors that may affect T cell response at the site of T cell recognition

MHC binding site (agretope) present on peptide
Affinity of agretope-MHC interaction
Secondary structure of peptide
T cell epitope present on peptide
Existence and extent of T cell repertoire

Factors Distant from the Site of T Cell Recognition: Aleatory Combinations in Immunodominance

Despite the importance of the site-related factors in determining the boundaries of response, a variety of aleatory effects are paramount in establishing dominance (*aleatory*, from the Latin stem meaning gambler, having connotations of both unpredictability/chance and dependence upon a contingent event). In table 3 are listed several of the possible influences that can affect the hierarchy of determinant response to a complex antigen, or in reference to a particular antigenic determinant, can alter the response to it, even though they are distant and distinct on the molecule. In this sense, the *molecular context* of a determinant will very directly affect the outcome of response, perhaps more than the nature of the potential determinant itself. These major contextual features of the architecture of the molecule, and their relationships to such aspects as the effectiveness of suppressor T cells in abrogating all responses, or the particular pattern of binding sites available on the MHC molecules in that haplotype, are aleatory in nature but will be the primary features that define the quality of the output, the program of the concert.

Regulatory T Cells Directed against Other Determinants

The idea that specific determinants on a protein antigen might be addressed to suppressor T cells and others to helper T cells was first presented in regard to the GZ molecule [29]. Actually, like keyhole-limpet hemocyanin (KLH), GZ is immunogenic in H-2^k strains and induces a strong response; however, both of these large protein antigens also concomitantly induce suppressor T cells.

We were studying the T and B cell responses to the lysozymes at the same time [30] and it was tempting to speculate that the reason for the unresponsiveness in certain H-2^b mouse strains such as C57BL/6 and A.BY was the coexistence of SD which nullified a response that otherwise would have taken place, fostered by HD. Later, it was learned that, indeed, a determinant at the N terminus of certain lysozymes (chicken, quail, guinea

Table 3. Factors that may affect T cell response related to features distant from T cell recognition site

Suppression: suppressor T cells directed against a distant determinant nullify reponse to HD
Receptor shielding: B cell paratope protects epitope and prevents nearby T cell determinants from being efficiently presented
Degree of access to T cell determinant: route to determinant in formidable, guarded by Scylla and Charybdis; Scylla: distant parts of native antigen affect access to determinant; Charybdis: nonrevelant Ia molecule preemptively binds another determinant

hen) induces suppressor T cells and was at least one critical feature contributing to the genetic unresponsiveness in these strains to HEL. Other lysozymes, such as those of the ring-necked pheasant (REL) and turkey, possess a tyrosine rather than phenylalanine at residue 3 of the molecule which is not consonant with suppressor T cell induction, and therefore these lysozymes are immunogenic in such H-2^b strains. Other complexities, presumably related to antigen presentation or to the presence of sufficient accessory stimulatory factors ('signal 2'), coded for by gene(s) on chromosome 2 [31, 32], also influence the level of responsiveness: thus, certain H-2^b strains such as C3H.SW, C57L and BALB.B produce a proliferative and antibody response to HEL, despite the existence of suppressor T cells.

Returning to the GZ system, the situation is somewhat different from HEL in that the tetrameric GZ molecule is more than 30 times as large as HEL. Therefore, it can be asked whether there is a high likelihood that suppressor T cells directed against a single determinant would be able to abolish the response to the rest of the molecule. Krzych et al. [33] and Shivakumar et al. [34] have addressed this question and the general conclusion is that, as expected from the fact that the CBA/J strain is a responder to GZ, there must be some helper T cells which are not susceptible to the activity of the suppressor T cells. A detailed analysis has shown that there is a clear propinquity effect – that SD and HD must be relatively close, probably about 50 amino acids away. In addition, it is clear that there are more SD than are apparent from a hasty study. In our experiments, which all had an antihapten (fluorescein) readout, it is evident that in order to specify an SD it is necessary to have a nearby helper T–B collaborative system functioning; thus, as more HD are identified, additional SD emerge from obscurity. An elegant study in a different system [35], again with 3 distinct functional antigenic elements, also revealed this interdependence.

The major secondary conclusion arising from the fact that suppressor T cells have a circumscribed hegemony is that if the *dominant* helper T cell response falls within this domain there very well may be complete unresponsiveness to the antigen. More often, at least one of the codominant HD on a very large antigen such as KLH or GZ lies outside of a nearby suppressor T cell domain, and this results in responsiveness. If it is true that a molecule can be represented as a mosaic of BD, HD and SD (in fact, in descending order of frequency), even on small antigens, it will be unpredictable whether the mere existence of an SD will insure nonresponsiveness. Actually, the responding H-2^b strains to lysozyme [31, 32] show that the delicate balance model may be closer to the natural situation.

Preferential T Cell–B Cell Partnerships

Soon after the demonstration that there was T and B cell collaboration in the immune response to carriers and haptens [36, 37], efforts were made to prove that, indeed, the same relationship held between the 'T' and 'B' determinants on any protein antigen [38–40]. Although this question was readily answered in the affirmative, the more difficult problem to solve was whether any determinant could act in both a T and B capacity. This was a premature question in a sense, because the true nature of T cell recognition would only be worked out a decade or so later. Nevertheless, it was possible to ask one of the facets of that question: can the same determinant be used for recognition by both T and B cells in a particular encounter? If not, or even if it *were* possible, is there an optimal distance between the T cell determinant and the B cell epitope, and are there preferential partnerships between such T and B cells?

A variety of answers and approaches have been used over the intervening years and those interested in the problem should consult the references mentioned in these paragraphs as well as the review by Berzofsky [41]. The framework for the problem lies in the realization that the epitope buried in the B cell receptor has, at least in its native conformation, strong affinity at various subsites to receptor residues and, therefore, occupies a special niche in the subsequent processing of antigen. Either the epitope proper is protected by the immunoglobulin active site, and never revealed to MHC molecules for presentation, or, at the opposite extreme, the epitope is protected and thereby readied for special delivery to class II molecules in the endosome. To summarize the solutions to this quandary, it appears that the latter alternative above is clearly not the favored route for delivery of processed agretope/T cell epitope to the MHC and that there may very well be a zone of preferential presentation of T cell determinants to the MHC by the antigen-immunoglobulin complex: this zone is probably close to the B cell epitope, at least in the three-dimensional initial form of the antigen. An estimate of the optimal distance between T and B epitopes was first made by Goodman's group [42, 43] who created synthetic antigens containing variable-length proline linkers.

In the GZ system, the starting molecule is rather large and was predicted to be a good prototype for searching for preferential partnerships, since it might be expected to be processed early, even within the immunoglobulin receptor, into smaller chunks that could serve as the substrate for the delivery to the class II molecule for presentation to the T cell. Thus, in 1985, Manca et al. [44] demonstrated differential help in the GZ system using various cyanogen bromide peptides to prime T cells. Preferential partners could be identified between certain T cells and the B cells that they activated, as measured by their ability to protect native, or activate mutant, forms of the enzyme. Finally, using different monoclonal antibodies, binding to GZ in GZ-monoclonal antibody complexes, as surrogate GZ-receptor complexes, Manca et al. [45] showed that only certain members of a panel of GZ-specific T hybridomas were activated by particular complexes.

With the smaller lysozyme molecule, Cecka et al. [46] have shown a shift in antibody specificity accompanying restriction of the available T cell repertoire in rabbits. Another example of favoritism was established with trinitrophenyl (TNP) derivatives of HEL at positions 33 and 96. The 34–54 lysozyme peptide raised T cells that distinguished between 96-TNP-HEL and 33-TNP-HEL in collaboration with B cells in the A/J mouse [47]. Most recently, it has been shown that determinant preferences in the relationship between lysozyme-specific T and B cells exist even in a totally in vivo system [48]. In another small antigen system, Ozaki and Berzofsky [49] showed that with myoglobin, constraints exist in collaboration between B and T cells specific for an overlapping determinant, confirming earlier studies with lysozyme [46].

At their essence, these intramolecular effects displayed between T and B cell epitopes involve a type of reciprocity, a term usefully enlisted by Berzofsky [50] to underline the fact that, although the T cell provides the help for the B cell, the latter provides the needed determinant for the T cell, and that these are interdependent quantities. Another probable corollary is that both T and B cell epitope must be present on the same antigenic fragment at the time of transfer of the determinant complex from the immunoglobulin active site to the MHC active site. In the next sections we will return to this crucial aspect of position in the determinant array that constitutes an antigen.

Interference with Access and Availability to a Determinant

In the current paradigm of antigen processing and presentation, mentioned earlier, immunodominance of determinants is simply a matter of the coexistence of agretope and MHC binding site and the energy of interaction between them. This model has no aleatory features, because the original position of the determinant within the molecule has no significance. Dominance simply becomes a predictable outcome of the laws of mass action.

However, the facts demand a consideration of molecular position, in particular the idea that residues distant from a potential site of T cell recognition can influence whether that site will really be utilized as a T cell determinant or not. 'Distant' here means reasonably far away on the molecule, and not the flanking residues near the determinant that can influence approach and docking to the MHC site [51], or the conformation of the determinant [52] and, therefore, its complementarity to the site. It must be recalled that usually, in the context of the whole-animal experiments where the subject receives a rather limited amount of a native antigen (at least compared to the culture well where its concentration is roughly 10 m*M*), what results from the encounter is the activation of a limited number of T cells, the dominant set. But what is dominant for the H-2^s goose is nondominant for the H-2^d gander!

Thus, what we must seek in explanation is strictly an MHC effect that leads to predominance of a single determinant in the native molecule *at the expense of others*. As a rule, any of the subdominant determinants would be potentially able to induce a vigorous antipeptide T cell response if they could be separated from their intramolecular neighbor determinants. In the next two sections, the Scylla and Charybdis of antigen handling will be confronted: the shielding of a determinant resulting in lack of access of the determinant to the MHC and the possible competition among MHC restriction elements for various determinants on the same antigenic molecule.

The Scylla Effect – Distractions in Antigen Processing and Presentation. En route to being processed and presented to ambient T cells, a specific, potential T cell determinant is clearly dependent on the nature of the neighboring portions of the antigenic molecule as to whether it will ever achieve its position in the MHC antigen-binding groove. In a sense, the most available agretopes on the antigen molecule act as Scylla, the beautiful sea nymph who metamorphosed into a sea monster causing distracted, errant sea captains to smash into the huge rock that now represents her. In order for determinants on HEL to have access to the MHC, this tightly wound molecule must at least be partially unfolded to reveal its agretopes: if processing of HEL is prevented, the antigen is not immunogenic [53–55]. (Interestingly, lysozyme is even resistant to tryptic cleavage until it is nicked or partially reduced [56].) During the process of unfolding, it can be argued that the first agretope to be revealed will bind to a complementary restriction element. If the agretope-desetope interaction is strong enough, it may be that the initially bound determinant will eventually be dominant. In any event, it is conceived that this initial binding will decisively affect the subsequent pathway of processing, perhaps favoring alternative pathways, protecting some sites from further cleavage by proteolytic enzymes, and generally leading to a different assortment of end products from that ordinarily produced in the absence of MHC class II molecules.

The evidence suggestive of this view has been presented and summarized elsewhere in extenso [57–60] but I will just review two experimental examples here.

(1) *Heterocliticity.* In the H-2^b mouse, all T cell clones directed to HEL are heteroclitic for the closely related REL, responding to REL at 50–100 times lower concentrations than to HEL. The fascinating feature of this effect is that when the N and C termini of the molecules are removed, leaving a large core of 93 amino acids (against which all of the clones are directed, in any case), the heterocliticity disappears. Thus, even for a clone specific for 81–96/A^b, the amino or carboxyl terminus exerts a substantial effect at a distance. The effect was interpreted as above, supposing that the ends of the molecule are crucial for some function in antigen handling, and exert a crucial influence on the pathways of processing leading to the production of determinants within the molecule [57].

(2) *Context.* T cells will be activated to specific determinants depending on the nature of the starting material. Accordingly, in the B6 mouse immunized with peptide 74–96 of HEL, clones of 74–90 and 81–96 specificity arise; however, the former are completely absent when cyanogen bromide fragment 13–105 is the immunogen, and the latter are absent when HEL is the immunogen. This striking result holds true for each of more than 50 clones in each of the two categories, as well as in fresh populations from lymph nodes. Evidently, enzymatic attack will differ greatly as a function of available and susceptible amino acid residues, and certain products of processing can only arise if conditions are favorable. This conclusion was also supported from a different direction, as Puri and Factorovich [61] have demonstrated that specific proteolytic enzyme inhibitors can prevent the utilization of particular determinants of a protein.

From this perspective, whether a particular determinant will ever have a chance to bind to the desetope site on an MHC molecule is an aleatory outcome of events that have little to do with the constitution of the determinant per se, but are consequences of molecular architecture, the characteristics of neighboring or even distant determinants or nondeterminants that dictate the disposition of the molecule when it enters the antigen-presenting cell. One competitive way in which distant determinants can play a decisive role is illustrated in the next section.

The Charybdis Effect – Aggressive Preemption by Other Restriction Elements. If the distant determinant happens to be the first to be uncovered, and has a reasonably strong affinity for the same *or another* restriction element, there will be a resultant competitive interference. In an attempt to establish whether there was functional interference even between determinants restricted to different MHC molecules, the H-2^d proliferative T cell response to HEL was studied. In this haplotype, recognition of HEL peptide p106–116 is restricted to E^d and, upon immunization with native HEL in strains displaying both an E^d and an A^d molecule, the response to this peptide is strongly dominant [62]. However, in such strains as B10.GD or D2.GD, in which the E^d molecule is not present on the surface of the cell, otherwise obscured responses restricted by A^d become dominant. Thus, a strong response to p20–35 is expressed after HEL priming, dominant over that to p116–129 in these latter strains.

The interpretation that the E^d MHC molecule captures the unfolding molecule which bears both E^d and A^d determinants, and thus prevents the A^d-restricted determinants from ready access to a high-affinity site for their presentation, implies that the capture process simultaneously includes an element of destruction for those other determinants. One apparent test for this model was a comparison between immunization of A^d- and E^d-bearing strains with peptide 106–129 versus a mixture of the peptides 106–116 and 116–129. Indeed in preliminary experiments, responses to the subdominant peptide could be obtained, but only if it were physically separate from the dominant peptide; when joined, only T cells specific for 106–116 were obtained. More work has to be done to examine this situation to see whether hindering flanking residues that do not constitute the agretypic core of 106–116 are responsible for the inability of 116–129 to gain access to the A^d restriction element.

It has been demonstrated previously that peptides using the same restriction element can compete, even in vivo, at the desetope site on the MHC molecule [63]: in these instances, the higher-affinity interaction should win out and determine dominance. However, the more usual competition probably occurs between determinants while they are still connected by the rest of the molecule. Through this intramolecular competition, aleatory effects will abound, as the hierarchy of determinants will be a consequence of that particular mix of competitive determinants, proteolytic enzymes and hindering structures, as well as the previously mentioned vagaries of B cell memory and T cell suppression.

From the foregoing, it might be expected that a distinct hierarchical pattern of dominance to an antigenic molecule would be a rare event indeed. This is not the case, since once the given molecule has been selected by the investigator, its architectonics will establish the hierarchy with respect to a given MHC haplotype. In fact, in cases where few determinants exist on a small molecule, a quite reproducible dominance occurs, and certain cryptic potential determinants reproducibly fail to induce T cells unless they are withdrawn from the molecule and injected as peptides. Even with very large molecules such as GZ, the choice of assay system circumscribes the dominance relationships and can lead to apparent dominance in a selected region of GZ. However, there are cases in which there is an abundance of codominant determinants. As an example, the $H\text{-}2^k$ haplotype can respond in some way to at least ten determinants on HEL [64].

In this special instance, Gammon et al. [65] have studied the frequency with which certain dominant determinants are used in different individual mice. The result represents aleatory variation of a second order: individuals 'select' a particular pattern of determinant preference and many patterns are demonstrable [65]. Additional variability arises from in vitro effects in that if T cell lines are grown from separate mice, certain clones, and clearly not the same ones, acquire dominance after long-term growth in vitro. It is clear that to arrive at a conclusion about dominance from the clonal specificity pattern of T cell hybridomas prepared from a long-term line is hazardous.

Returning to our initial musical analogy, we have provided some evidence for the aleatory nature of 'molecular concert programs'. It is hoped that soon we will understand on showing up at the performance why the conductor happened to choose Bartok rather than Brahms.

References

1 Wicker, L.S.; Benjamin, C.D.; Miller, A.; Sercarz, E.E.: Immunodominant protein epitopes. II. The primary antibody response to hen egg white lysozyme required and focuses upon a unique N-terminal epitope. Eur. J. Immunol. *14:* 447–453 (1984).

2 Sercarz, E.: Epitypic/idiotypic dominance as an evolutionary answer to the intercellular communication problem; in Sercarz, Celada, Mitchison, Tada, The semiotics of cellular communication in the immune system, pp. 315–326 (Springer, Heidelberg 1988).

3 Sercarz, E.; Araneo, B.; Benjamin, C.D.; Harvey, M.; Metzger, D.; Miller, A.; Wicker, L.; Yowell, R.: The design of regulatory circuitry: predominant idiotypy and the idea of regulatory parsimony: in Bona, Kohler, Immune networks. Ann. N.Y. Acad. Sci. *418:* 198–205 (1983).

4 Benjamin, D.C.; Berzofsky, J.A.; East, I.J.; Gurd, F.R.N.; Hannum, C.; Leach, S.J.; Margoliash, E.; Michael, J.G.; Miller, A.; Prager, E.M.; Reichlin, M.; Sercarz, E.E.; Smith-Gill, S.J.; Todd, P.E.; Wilson, A.C.: The antigenic structure of proteins: a reappraisal. Annu. Rev. Immunol. *2:* 67–101 (1984).

5 Adorini, L.; Harvey, M. A.; Miller, A.; Sercarz, E.E.: The fine specificity of regulatory T cells. II. Suppressor and helper T cells are induced by different regions of hen egg-white lysozyme (HEL) in a genetically nonresponder mouse strain. J. exp. Med. *150:* 293–306 (1979).

6 Krzych, U.; Fowler, A.; Miller, A.; Sercarz, E.E.: Helper and suppressor T cells are induced by nonoverlapping determinants on the large protein antigen, β-galactosidase. FASEB J. *2:* 141–144 (1988).

7 Maizels, R.; Clarke, J.; Harvey, M.; Miller, A.; Sercarz, E.E.: Epitope specificity of the T cell proliferative response to lysozyme: T proliferative cells react predominantly to different determinants from those recognized by B cells. Eur. J. Immunol. *10:* 509–515 (1980).

8 Gershon, R.K.: T cell regulation: second law of thymodynamics; in Sercarz, Williamson, Fox, The immune system: genes, receptors, signals, p. 471–484 (Acad. Press, New York 1974).

9 Manca, F.; Clarke, J.A.; Sercarz, E.E.; Miller, A.: T cells with differing specificity exist for a single determinant on lysozyme; in Pierce, Cullen, Schwartz, Kapp, Shreffler, 5th Ir Gene Symp. Ir genes: past, present and future, pp. 311–315 (Humana Press, Clifton 1983).

10 Katz, M.E.; Miller, A.; Krzych, U.; Wicker, L.; Maizels, R.; Clarke, J.; Shastri, N.; Oki, A.; Sercarz, E.E.: Hierarchical relationships among epitopes on protein antigens are actually presented in a particular haplotype; in Pierce, Cullen, Schwartz, Kapp, Shreffler, 5th Ir Gene Symp. Ir genes: past, present and future, Ibid. pp. 317–323 (Humana Press, Clifton 1983).

11 Manca, F.; Clarke, J.; Shastri, N.; Miller, A.; Sercarz, E.E.: A limited region within hen eggwhite lysozyme serves as the focus for a diversity of T cell clones. J. Immun. *133:* 2075–2078 (1984).

12 Heber-Katz, E.; Hansburg, D.; Schwartz, R.H.: The Ia molecule of the antigen-presenting cell plays a critical role in immune response gene regulation of T cell activation. J. mol. cell. Immunol. *1:* 3–14 (1983).

13 Allen, P.M.; McKean, D.J.; Beck, B.N.; Sheffield, J.; Glimcher, L.H.: Direct evidence that a class II molecule and a simple globular protein generate multiple determinants. J. exp. Med. *162:* 1264–1274 (1985).

14 Shastri, N.; Oki, A.; Miller, A.; Sercarz, E.E.: Distinct recognition phenotypes exist for T cell clones specific for small peptide regions of proteins: implications for the mechanisms underlying MHC-restricted antigen recognition and clonal deletion models of immune response gene defects. J. exp. Med. *162:* 332–345 (1985).

15 Shimonkevitz, R.; Colon, S.; Kappler, J.W.; Marrack, P.; Grey, H.M.: Antigen recognition by H-2-restricted T cells. II. A tryptic ovalbumin peptide that substitutes for processed antigen. J.Immun. *133:* 2067–2074 (1984).

16 Ogasawara, K.; Maloy, W.; Schwartz, R.H.: Failure to find holes in the T cell repertoire. Nature *325:* 450 (1987).

17 Acha-Orbea, H.; Mitchell, D.J.; Timmermann, L.; Wraith, D.C.; Tausch, G.S.; Waldor, M.K.; Zamvil, S.S.; McDevitt, H.O.; Steinman, L.: Limited heterogeneity of T cell receptors from lymphocytes mediating autoimmune encephalomyelitis allows specific immune intervention. Cell *54:* 263–273 (1988).

18 Zamvil, S.S.; Mitchell, D.J.; Moore, A.C.; Kitamura, K.; Steinman, L.; Rothbard, J.B.: T-cell epitope of the autoantigen myelin basic protein that induces encephalomyelitis. Nature *324:* 258–260 (1986).

19 Urban, J.L.; Kumar, V.; Kono, D.H.; Gomez, C.; Horvath, S.J.; Clayton, J.; Ando, D.G.; Sercarz, E.E.; Hood, L.: Restricted use of T cell receptor V genes in murine autoimmune encephalomyelitis raises possibilities for antibody therapy. Cell *54:* 577–592 (1988).

20 Sette, A.; Buus, S.; Grey, H.: Molecular basis and functional relevance of peptide-Ia interactions; in Smith-Gill, Sercarz, The immune response to structurally defined proteins: the lysozyme model (Adenine Press, New York 1989).

21 Apple, R.; Clarke, J.; Cogswell, J.; Gammon, G.; Katz, M.E.; Krzych, U.; Maizels, R.; Manca, F.; Miller, A.; Nasseri, S.; Oki, A.; Wilbur, S.; Sercarz, E.E.: The causes and consequences of immunodominance at the T cell level; in Smith-Gill, Sercarz, The immune response to structurally defined proteins: the lysozyme model (Adenine Press, New York 1989).

22 Buus, S.; Sette, A.; Colon, S.M.; Miles, C.; Grey, H.M.: The relation between major histocompatibility complex (MHC) restriction and the capacity of Ia to bind immunogenic peptides. Science *235:* 1353–1358 (1987).

23 Kappler, J.W.; Roehm, N.; Marrack, P.: T cell tolerance by clonal elimination in the thymus. Cell *49:* 273–280 (1987).

24 Kappler, J.W.; Staerz, U.D.; White, J.; Marrack P.: Self-tolerance eliminates T cells specific for Mls-modified products of the major histocompatibility complex. Nature *332:* 35–40 (1988).

25 McDonald, H.R.; Schneider, R.; Lees, R.K.; Howe, R.C.; Acha-Orbea, H.; Festenstein, H.; Zinkernagel, R.M.; Hengartner, H.: T-cell receptor Vβ use predicts reactivity and tolerance to Mls^a-encoded antigens. Nature *332:* 40–45 (1988).

26 White, J.; Herman, A.; Pullen, A.M.; Kubo, R.; Kappler, J.W.; Marrack, P.: The Vβ-specific superantigen staphylococcal enterotoxin B: stimulation of mature T cells and clonal deletion in neonatal mice. Cell *56:* 27–35 (1989).

27 Guillet, J.-G.; Lai, M.Z.; Briner, T.J.; Buus, S.; Sette, A.; Grey, H.M.; Smith, J.A.; Gefter, M.L.: Immunological self, nonself discrimination. Science *235:* 865–870 (1987).

28 Sette, A.; Buus, S.; Colon, S.; Smith, J.A.; Miles, C.; Grey, H.M.: Structural characteristics of an antigen required for its interaction with Ia and recognition by T cells. Nature *328:* 395–399 (1987).

29 Sercarz, E.E.; Corenzwit, D.T.; Eardley, D.E.; Morris, K.M.: Suppressive versus helper effects in carrier priming; in Singhal, Sinclair, Suppressor cells in immunity, p. 19 (University of Western Ontario Press, London, Ont. 1975).

30 Hill, S.; Sercarz, E.E.: Fine specificity of an immune response gene for the gallinaceous lysozymes. Eur. J. Immunol. *5:* 317–324 (1975).

31 Sadegh-Nasseri, S.; Kipp, D.E.; Taylor, B.A.; Miller, A.; Sercarz, E.E.: Selective reversal of H-2 linked genetic unresponsiveness to lysozymes. I. Non-H-2 gene(s) closely linked to the *Ir-2* locus on chromosome 2 permit(s) an anti-lysozyme response in $H\text{-}2^b$ mice. Immunogenetics *20:* 535–546 (1984).

32 Sadegh-Nasseri, S.; Dessi, V.; Sercarz, E.E.: Selective reversal of H-2 linked genetic unresponsiveness to lysozymes. II. Alteration in the T-helper/T-suppressor balance owing to gene(s) linked to Ir-2 leads to responsiveness in BALB.B. Eur. J. Immunol. *16:* 486–492 (1986).

33 Krzych, U.; Fowler, A.V.; Sercarz, E.E.: Repertoire of T cells directed against a large protein antigen, β-galactosidase. II. Only certain T helper or T suppressor cells are relevant in particular regulatory interactions. J. exp. Med. *162:* 311–323 (1985).

34 Shivakumar, S.; Sercarz, E.E.; Krzych, U.: The molecular context of determinants within the priming antigen establishes a hierarchy of T cell induction: T cell specificities induced by peptides of β-galactosidase versus the whole antigen. Eur. J. Immunol. (in press, 1989).

35 Asano, Y.; Hodes, R.J.: T cell regulation of B cell activation: an antigen-mediated tripartite interaction of Ts cells, Th cells, and B cells is required for suppression. J. Immun. *133:* 2864–2867 (1984).

36 Mitchison, N.A.: The carrier effect in the secondary response to hapten-protein conjugates. II. Cellular cooperation. Eur. J. Immunol. *1:* 18 (1971).

37 Katz, D.H.; Paul, W.E.; Goidl, E.A.; Benacerraf, B.: Carrier function in anti-hapten immune responses. I. Enhancement of primary and secondary anti-hapten antibody responses by carrier preimmunization. J. exp. Med. *132:* 261 (1970).

38 Rajewsky, K.; Schirrmacher, V.; Nase, S.; Jerne, N. K.: The requirement for more than one antigenic determinant for immunogenicity. J. exp. Med. *129:* 1131 (1969).

39 Bonavida, B.; Sercarz, E.E.: Structural basis for immune recognition of lysozymes. II. Reactive but nonimmunogenic epitopes on hen egg-white lysozyme. Eur. J. Immunol. *1:* 166 (1971).

40 Berzofsky, J.A.; Schechter, A.N.; Shearer, G.M.; Sachs, D.H.: Genetic control of the immune response to staphylococcal nuclease. III. Time-course and correlation between the response to native nuclease and the response to its polypeptide fragments. J. exp. Med. *145:* 111 (1977).

41 Berzofsky, J.A.: Ir genes: antigen-specific genetic regulation of the immune responses; in Sela, M., The antigens (Academic Press, New York 1987).
42 Bush, M.E.; Alkan, S.S.; Nitecki, D.E.; Goodman, J.W.: Antigen recognition and the immune response: 'self-help' with symmetrical bifunctional antigen molecules. J. exp. Med. *136:* 1478–1483 (1972).
43 Fong, S.; Nitecki, D.E.; Cook, R.M.; Goodman, J.W.: Spatial requirements between haptenic and carrier determinants for T-dependent antibody responses. J. exp. Med. *148:* 817–822 (1978).
44 Manca, F.; Kunkl, A.; Fenoglio, D.; Fowler, A.; Sercarz, E.E.; Celada, F.: Constraints in T-B cooperation related to epitope topology on *E. coli* β-galactosidase. I. The fine specificity of T cells dictates the fine specificity of antibodies directed to conformation-dependent determinants. Eur. J. Immunol. *15:* 345–350 (1985).
45 Manca, F.; Fenoglio, D.; Kunkl, A.; Cambiaggi, C.; Sasso, M.; Celada, F.: Differential activation of T cell clones stimulated by macrophages exposed to antigen complexed with monoclonal antibodies: a possible influence of paratope specificity on the mode of antigen processing. J. Immun. *140:* 2893–2898 (1988).
46 Cecka, J.M.; Stratton, J.A.; Miller, A.; Sercarz, E.E.: Structural aspects of immune recognition of the lysozymes. III. T-cell specificity restriction and its consequences for antibody specificity. Eur. J. Immunol. *6:* 639–646 (1976).
47 Hirayama, A.; Dohi, Y.; Takagaki, Y.; Fujio, H.; Amano, T.: Structural relationships between carrier epitopes and antigenic epitopes on hen egg-white lysozyme. Immunology *46:* 145–154 (1982).
48 Palmer, M.; Sercarz, E.: Determinant preferences in the relationship between T and B cells specific for lysozyme; in Smith-Gill, Sercarz, The immune response to structurally defined proteins: the lysozyme model (Adenine Press, New York 1989).
49 Ozaki, S.; Berzofsky, J.A.: Antibody conjugates mimic specific B cell presentation of antigen: relationship between T and B cell specificity. J. Immun. *12:* 4133–4142 (1987).
50 Berzofsky, J.A.: T-B reciprocity: an Ia restricted epitope-specific circuit regulates T cell-B cell interaction and antibody specificity. Surv. immunol. Res. *2:* 223 (1983).
51 Brett, S.J.; Cease, K.B.; Berzofsky, J.A.: Influences of antigen processing on the expression of the T cell repertoire: evidence for MHC-specific hindering structures on the products of processing. J. exp. Med. *168:* 357 (1988).
52 Boyer, M.; Novak, Z.; Fotedar, A.; Singh, B.: Contribution of antigen processing to the recognition of a synthetic peptide antigen by specific T cell hybridomas. J. mol. Rec. *1:* 99–106 (1988).
53 Shastri, N.; Miller, A.; Sercarz, E.E.: The interpretation of T cell specificity: the role of antigen processing by antigen presenting cells; in Cantor, Chess, Sercarz, Regulation of the immune system, pp. 153–161 (Liss, New York 1984).
54 Allen, P.M.; Unanue, E.R.: Differential requirements for antigen processing by macrophages for lysozyme-specific T hybridomas. J. Immun. *132:* 1077–1079 (1984).
55 Lorenz, R.G.; Allen, P.M.: Direct evidence for functional self-protein/Ia-molecule complexes in vivo. Proc. natn. Acad. Sci. USA *35:* 5220–5223 (1988).
56 Bonavida, B.; Miller, A.; Sercarz, E.E.: Structural basis for immune recognition of lysozyme. I. Comparison of native and cyanogen-bromide treated lysozyme. Biochemistry *8:* 989 (1969).
57 Shastri, N.; Miller, A.; Sercarz, E.E.: The expressed T cell repertoire is hierarchical: the precise focus of lysozyme-specific T cell clones is dependent upon the structure of the immunogen. J. mol. cell Immunol. *1:* 369–377 (1985).
58 Shastri, N.; Miller, A.; Sercarz, E.E.: Amino acid residues distinct from the determinant

region can profoundly affect activation of T cell clones by related antigens. J. Immun. *136:* 371–376 (1986).
59 Shastri, N.; Gammon, G.; Horvath, S.; Miller, A.; Sercarz, E.E.: The choice between two distinct T cell determinants within a 23 amino acid region of lysozyme depends upon structure of the immunogen. J. Immun. *137:* 911–915 (1986).
60 Sercarz, E.; Wilbur, S.; Sadegh-Nasseri, S.; Miller, A.; Manca, F.; Gammon, G.; Shastri, N.: The molecular context of a determinant influences its dominant expression in a T cell response hierarchy through 'fine processing'. Prog. Immunol. *6:* 227–237 (1986).
61 Puri, J.; Factorovich, Y.: Selective inhibition of antigen presentation to cloned T cells by protease inhibitors. J. Immun. *14:* 3313–3317 (1988).
62 Cogswell, J.P.; Gammon, G.; Wilbur, S.; Shastri, N.; Miller, A.; Sercarz, E.E.: Ia dependent selection of agretopes on the partially unfolded chicken lysozyme molecule affects subsequent processing pathways and the dominance of T cell determinants; in Schook, Antigen presenting cells, pp. 115–126 (Liss, New York 1988).
63 Adorini, L.; Muller, S.; Cardinaux, F.; Lehmann, P.; Falcioni, F.; Nagy, Z.: In vivo competition between self peptides and foreign antigens in T cell activation. Nature *334:* 623 (1988).
64 Adorini, L.; Appella, E.; Doria, G.; Nagy, Z.A.: Mechanisms influencing the immunodominance of T cell determinants. J. exp. Med. *168:* 2091–2104 (1988).
65 Gammon, G.; Klotz, J.; Ando, D.; Sercarz, E.: The T cell repertoire to a multideterminant antigen: heterogeneity in the specificity of response among individuals of the same inbred mouse strain (submitted, 1989).
66 Martinez-A., C.; Coutinho, A.; Bandeira, A.; de la Hera, A.; Toribio, M.; Marcos, M.A.R.; Pereira, P.: Sporadic idiotypic cross-reactivities between antibodies and T helper cells: one example of aleatory expression of T cell idiotypes. J. mol. cell. Immunol. *3:* 21–28 (1987).

Eli E. Sercarz, PhD, Department of Microbiology, University of California,
Los Angeles, CA 90024 (USA)

Subject Index